The Smart Woman's Guide to Breast Cancer

The Functional Medicine Approach That Will Free You From Your Diagnosis

By Jenn Simmons, MD

The Smart Woman's Guide to Breast Cancer

The Functional Medicine Approach That Will Free You From Your Diagnosis

Jenn Simmons, MD

Copyright © 2024

All Rights Reserved.

For more information: www.realhealthmd.com

Cover Design: Rachael Pollack

ISBN: 9798324741402

TABLE OF CONTENTS

Foreword by Mark Hyman, MD

Breast cancer is a journey that no woman wants to embark on. Yet, in The Smart Woman's Guide to Breast Cancer, an illuminating and profoundly impactful path is carved for those who find themselves navigating this challenging terrain. This book is more than a guide; it is a beacon of hope and a testament to the power of understanding, insight, empowerment, intuition, and healing from a functional medicine perspective.

As someone deeply committed to transforming healthcare and understanding the root causes of disease, I find the approach of this book to be revolutionary. It aligns with the foundational belief that to truly heal, we must look beyond the conventional treatment paradigms of surgery, chemotherapy, and radiation, which often address only the symptoms, not the cause. This book empowers women to dive deep into the "why" of their diagnosis, offering a path to understanding their body's signals and what breast health truly means in the context of overall health.

What makes this book stand out is its commitment to empowering women with knowledge and tools to take control of their health journey. It does not shy away from the complexities of breast cancer, nor does it offer oversimplified solutions. Instead, it provides a clear, insightful, and actionable guide that respects the intelligence of its readers.

For any woman facing a breast cancer diagnosis, The Smart Woman's Guide to Breast Cancer is a must-read. It offers not just hope, but a practical and scientifically grounded approach to healing. It's a reminder that your health journey is yours to navigate, and with the right knowledge and support, you can take control of your healing process. I commend Dr. Jenn Simmons for her dedication in the following pages to changing the narrative around breast cancer and for providing a resource that will undoubtedly transform lives.

— Mark Hyman, MD, Functional Medicine Physician, *Fifteen-time New York Times* Best Selling author, and internationally recognized leader, speaker, advocate, and educator in his field.

Praise for *The Smart Woman's Guide To Breast Cancer*

"Dr. Jenn Simmons has written an informative and practical guide for breast cancer patients. *The Smart Woman's Guide to Breast Cancer* will empower you with knowledge to help you understand the different types of the disease, the benefits and risks of various treatment options, the value of integrative functional medicine, and the evidence-based diet and lifestyle strategies that can increase your odds of survival. This book contains critical information that your breast cancer surgeon and oncologist will not tell you, and important questions that you must ask in order to make the best treatment decisions for you. Dr. Jenn Simmons is a brilliant and courageous physician and as a twenty-year holistic colon cancer survivor and patient advocate, I am thankful for the good work that she is doing to help her patients survive and thrive through breast cancer." — Chris Wark, ChrisBeatCancer.com

"Dr. Jenn Simmons' *The Smart Woman's Guide to Breast Cancer* is a powerful roadmap for transforming fear into empowerment. As a fellow advocate for taking control of your health, I'm thrilled to see a book that not only educates but also inspires action. Jenn's approach to using functional medicine to move beyond a diagnosis is a testament to her dedication and passion. This book is a must-read for anyone looking to navigate their healing journey with grace and knowledge." — JJ Virgin, *New York Times* Bestselling Author

"*The Smart Woman's Guide to Breast Cancer* is a true beacon of hope, blending the best of conventional and functional medicine. Dr. Jenn's expert guidance is a lifeline for navigating this common and complex disease. This book is a must-read for anyone who is determined to heal and thrive after a breast cancer diagnosis." — William W. Li, MD *New York Times* bestselling author of Eat to Beat Disease and Eat to Beat Your Diet

"Dr. Jenn Simmons' *The Smart Woman's Guide to Breast Cancer* is an essential, empowering resource. She combines the latest science with practical advice, guiding women through their journey with wisdom and compassion. A must- read for anyone touched by breast cancer." — Dr. Tom O'Bryan, world- renowned expert in the field of chronic disease and autoimmune disorders.

"Dr. Jenn Simmons' *The Smart Woman's Guide to Breast Cancer* is an indispensable guide that lights the way for women facing breast cancer. With her expert knowledge and compassionate approach, Dr. Jenn empowers women to become active participants in their healing. This book brilliantly combines functional medicine principles with practical advice, making it an essential tool for anyone looking to thrive beyond their diagnosis. A true masterpiece of hope and healing." — Dr. Kellyann Petrucci, *New York Times* Bestselling Author, Founder: Drkellyann.com

"As a breast cancer survivor as well as functional medicine physician and nutritionist, I am thrilled Dr. Jenn Simmons has written, The Smart Women's Guide To Breast Cancer. This book is an amazing resource for anyone who has breast cancer or who wants to prevent breast cancer. Dr. Jenn takes us beyond the treatment of the tumor to the critically important discussion about the terrain that the tumor is bathed in, showing us how we can shift our body into one where cancer is less likely to grow." — Elizabeth Boham, MD, MS, RD

INTRODUCTION

As you might imagine, my job as a breast surgeon required me to attend many continuing medical education conferences. One year, The American Society of Breast Surgeons' annual meeting was in Las Vegas. The meeting was held at Caesar's Palace, home to many fabulous headliners. I prefer to travel with my husband, but he wasn't available on this occasion due to his own work conflict, so I asked my mother to join me.

My parents live for their dog. As a result, they rarely travel and when they do it is solely to places that allow dogs. My parents don't have a sweet, cute, little dog. I didn't grow up with Poodles or Shih Tzus. We had German Shepherds. When I went to college, they were introduced to a new breed which would forever change their life. Their new breed of choice is the Chinese Shar-Pei—you know, the wrinkly dogs. The breed is fabulous to look at, but the personality leaves a lot to be desired. That coupled with their menacing appearance makes them a less-than-ideal travel companion.

My parents' favorite color of Shar-Pei is blue. They are gorgeous and the rarest of the breed, and therefore the most expensive. At the time of the conference, my parents had a Shar-Pei named RJ. As I anticipated, my mom asked if RJ could join us in Las Vegas. As RJ was a spectacle, and awesome to look at, he garnered a lot of attention. He was also as mean as a pit viper. Keep in mind, this was many years ago, long before people widely traveled with their dogs. This was not a conversation that I wanted to have with her. I did not want her to bring the dog and I didn't want to tell her that.

My mother is a woman that doesn't like to be told no. A renowned event planner, she is only familiar with being in charge. Over her long and successful career, she worked for the president of Caesar's International. I told my mother that I really thought it was best for her to leave the dog at home, but she could call Mark Juliano's office, then-President of the Caesars Palace Las Vegas, and ask him. I was relieved not to be responsible for making that decision and to avoid the potential negative fallout that I would have to surely endure in my saying no. She called Mr. Juliano's office and was told by his assistant that there were no dogs allowed. She reluctantly acquiesced.

A month later, we arrived at the hotel for the conference. We checked in, dropped our bags off at our room and went out to explore. If you're not familiar with Caesars Palace in Vegas, it is a mecca of shopping and entertainment.

My mother and I were walking through the hotel headed toward the Forum, perhaps the most phenomenal shopping mall ever, when my mother suddenly stopped and gasped as if something catastrophic had just happened. I turned to her, grabbed her arm, and said, "Mom, what's wrong?" She looked at me and angrily said:

"I thought you said there were no dogs allowed!"

I gazed around to look at what on earth she was talking about. She was right. She did see a dog in the hotel. Just ahead, there was a gentleman with an adorable little dog walking toward us.

"Mom, yes, you can have a dog. If you are ELTON JOHN!"

Often, we are so focused on one thing that we lose sight of what's around it, where it's coming from, or what it means. A breast cancer diagnosis is almost always a result of something. It does not exist alone and it is not a breast problem. By focusing on the breast alone, and not observing the landscape, we will always miss something. Most times, what we miss will be major. Like my mother focused on nothing but the dog, conventional medicine focuses on nothing but the tumor and everything else is unseen. I know this because I spent a long time in this space focused on the tumor alone.

As a conventional medical doctor, this is exactly what I was trained to do. I was trained to recognize a constellation of symptoms, give it a name, and then prescribe a standard treatment. If it is a benign tumor, cut it out. If it is cancer, cut it, drug it, and burn it. This standard plan worked well for most breast cancer in that it prevented it from returning. What it didn't work well for was the women housing the cancer. Life after breast cancer treatment was fraught with life-altering side effects, most of them negative. Some were even worse than breast cancer itself. When I was working as a breast surgeon, I couldn't see this. As my friend and mentor JJ Virgin tells me, it's hard to see the picture when you're in the frame. It took my own experience as a patient for me to see the truth: our medical system is broken. It is focused on the wrong thing. I wrote this book to shine light on a lesser known but far better path to health. It's time for all of us to prioritize our health, but we need to know how to do that. There is no opportunity for us to do that in the current system. What we have is a sick care system. What we need is a healthcare system. While we are waiting for that to happen, I wrote this book so that, like me, you can start to help heal yourself. No one is ever going to know you better than you know yourself. No one is ever going to care about you or for you as much as you and your loved ones do.

I hope you use this book to create a happy, healthy you, and so that your light shines on your family, your friends and your community. This book and the principles outlined in it can benefit everyone. As I always say, "Breast Health is Health," and by following what is recommended in this book, you can help yourself create healthy breasts, and a healthy heart, brain, gut, bones, muscles, joints, and skin.

I want to thank my family for their support. Without my husband, Albert, this would never have been possible. He has been my staunch supporter from day one. He has always encouraged me to play bigger. Albert, I think I have finally arrived at the place where you always knew I belonged. Thank you for convincing me to keep going and keep growing. I know that was a big lift. You are the strongest man I know.

I also want to thank my boys, Andrew and Will, for understanding that my work was important. I am sorry I missed so much. I hope that you can look back and just be proud that I set out to change the world, and I did.

Lastly, I want to thank LG, my dear friend, confidant, quintessential mother, and supreme provider of advice and guidance. You told me that I couldn't leave surgery at the age of fifty and start over. I don't get to tell you that often that you are wrong. Thank God I didn't listen to you this time. Love you so much though!

CHAPTER ONE - MY STORY

In March of 2017, my life changed on a dime. On this terrible Tuesday, I went from seemingly having it all to losing my health in an instant. At that time, I was a top doc, had a beautiful marriage and family, a vibrant social life, was active in lots of charitable organizations, did tons of public speaking, had TV and media appearances, and was a six-day-a-week athlete. By all accounts I was at the pinnacle of my personal and professional life. Then, on this day, I lost everything and my practically perfect world came crumbling down. I went from being invincible to not being able to finish a sentence without getting out of breath. I was unable to walk across the room or up a flight of stairs. I saw my doctor and three days later received my diagnosis:

Graves' Disease.

This sparked my exploration to heal myself. I didn't have any higher motivation other than to feel better—this journey was about me. Never did I think what I would learn would change the rest of my life and how I would eventually touch the lives of millions of people.

My healing journey began in a pretty unsuspecting place. My diagnosis left me frightened and confused. Other than traditional medicine, I had no idea where to turn. I ended up going to Dr. Google and asking, "How can I heal my thyroid?

Dr. Google intimated that my illness may have something to do with my diet. Like most physicians, my nutritional training was lacking, to say the least. After some searching, I discovered an online training program that I decided was a good place to start. Though I was skeptical, I was committed to getting what I could out of this program. I was sitting in one of the very first lectures when a tall, handsome man with a toothy grin walked on the stage and introduced himself as a functional medicine physician. At this point in my career I had been a physician for nearly twenty years. In all that time I had never heard of a functional medicine doctor, and if I'm being honest, I wondered what this quack was talking about.

This quack was Dr. Mark Hyman and he was about to change my life.

Dr. Mark Hyman is a New York Times best-selling author. He is the figurehead and leader of the functional medicine movement and, along with its founder, Dr. Jeffrey Bland, legitimizes functional medicine by approaching it scientifically. He is the former chair of the Department of Functional Medicine at the Cleveland Clinic where he now serves as one of their senior advisors. He has several TED talks, a Podcast (The Doctor's Farmacy), and has been instrumental in the creation of policies aimed at solving the world's food problems. I didn't know any of that at the time.

The concept that Dr. Hyman introduced to the audience that day was inflammation. He explained all the inflammatory stimuli in our environment and the impact that it was having on our health and well-being. As I sat there listening to him speak about functional medicine, I was struck with a lightning bolt of enlightenment. The way he was discussing the current state of affairs and what was happening in this country and with our medical system made everything suddenly made sense. I instantly saw my life's purpose. Immediately, it became clear not only why I was sick, but why my patients were sick. And it also became crystal clear what I needed to do to start to cure myself and my patients. What resonated so much with me, and what eventually led to my leaving surgery, was that he was talking about the root cause of disease. Our current medical system is entirely focused on disease—on the management of symptoms. It does not begin to address why the symptoms exist in the first place. It does not question what the symptoms are a sign of. In fact, our medical system is not really designed to heal. It's not designed to cure. It's designed for symptom management and the perpetuation of disease. This is best illustrated by The Tack Theory.[1]

It goes like this. If you have a tack in your foot, you can either:

A. Take a lot of aspirin to relieve the pain or,

B. Remove the tack from your foot.

What we are meant to learn here is that pain is the symptom of the problem, not the problem. The problem is the tack. Our medical system is entirely focused on the symptom. In the world of cancer, the tumor is the symptom.

All cancer treatments are directed at the tumor—the symptom.

Only the tumor is not the problem. The tumor is the symptom of the problem. When we direct all our "treatment" at the tumor, we ignore the reason why the cancer developed in the first place. Without addressing the cause, or the root of the problem, we can never "cure" the problem.

I don't really like to talk about curing cancer. That is because cancer is the symptom. There is no one thing that is going to cure cancer. Cancer happens when there is imbalance in the system. The only way to cure cancer is for us to be healthy. Health doesn't come from pills, potions, surgery, or treatments. Health happens when we do the things that drive health. And the medical system is not driving health.

We don't have a healthcare system, we have a sick care system. This is a major problem.

Do you know what makes a really good doctor in our conventional medical system? The brilliant diagnostician—the person that can name the disease and prescribe the "treatment." As medical students and physician trainees, we are taught to recognize a constellation of symptoms, give it a name, and then prescribe a procedure or a medicine or some sort of intervention aimed at the symptom.

---

[1] This is not my theory. I heard this from Dr Mark Hyman who I believe heard this from Dr. Jeffrey Bland. The who here is not as important as the what.

For example, let's say that you're having symptoms of reflux. You go to the gastroenterologist; they schedule you for an endoscopy. Maybe they do a pH probe. Maybe they don't even do that. Maybe they just put you on reflux medication: a proton pump inhibitor (PPI). H2 blockers. What they don't do is say, "Gee, I wonder why you're having heartburn? Could it be food sensitivity? Could it be stress? An infection? Low stomach acid? Weight gain? What else is going on?"

As physicians, we are not trained to ask these questions. We are trained to diagnose and prescribe. Unfortunately, in the case of acid blockers and PPIs, we are prescribing them way too often and using them for way too long. As a result, we are suppressing people's immune systems, increasing the likelihood that they will develop infections, interfering with their ability to nourish themselves, causing nutritional deficits, and ultimately making them vulnerable to developing cancer. PPIs were originally approved for short-term use (two to four weeks). Long-term use is only recommended in selected populations, but data indicates that long-term use accounts for most of the total use.[2] We have adopted this "if some is good, more must be better" mentality. This works great for big Pharma, but not so much for people, and we are all paying the price.

And what a price we're paying. The United States spends more on health care than any other country in the world, yet we rank 47th in life expectancy. Despite our "healthcare" spend, the US suffers the highest burden for chronic diseases and two times higher obesity rates than the Organisation for Economic Co-operation and Development (OECD) average. The US also has the highest rate of hospitalizations, the highest number of preventable diseases, and the highest rate of avoidable deaths. The US is rated number 35 out of 169 countries in overall citizen health. These numbers do not bode well for the quality of our medical system. Unfortunately, as the world becomes more Americanized, by following our practices and examples, they are losing their health too.

---

[2] Raghunath, A. S., C O'Moráin, and Ramona McLoughlin. 2005. "Review Article: The Long-term Use of Proton-pump Inhibitors." Alimentary Pharmacology & Therapeutics 22 (s1): 55–63. https://doi.org/10.1111/j.1365-2036.2005.02611.x.

It's time for a new perspective.

I remember the day I walked away from surgery like it was yesterday. I was holding office hours and a nineteen-year-old woman rolled into my office in a wheelchair pushed by her mother.

By coincidence, I had just met a woman named Dr. Terry Wahls. Dr. Wahls is an awe-inspiring physician who was diagnosed with primary progressive multiple sclerosis (MS) while she was the residency program director at the Iowa Veteran Affairs Medical Center where she practiced internal medicine. Hers was a very aggressive form of MS, and within three years she went from being a normal, high functioning woman to being confined to a zero-gravity wheelchair. This meant that she no longer had the strength to support her own body weight. She was let go by the hospital because she was incapable of performing her duties as a physician and an educator. This is someone who was deeply ingrained in the medical system. She had access to everything—every drug, clinical trial, anything that the traditional medical system had to offer. However, despite all that, her health continued to fail.

Desperate to find something that would at least slow her disease, she began searching. What she found was nothing short of astounding. In fact, the method that she eventually trademarked, The Wahls Protocol, not only saved her life, but has saved the lives of thousands of people that have adopted that protocol.

The young girl who entered my office that day had such advanced MS at nineteen that she couldn't walk the thirty feet from the elevator to the exam room. She was coming to me for a breast mass. I was a giddy school child that day, eager to share Dr. Wahls' story and infuse this girl and her mother with the hope that I truly believed would change the rest of her life. But, after two minutes of my speaking, she put her hand up, halted me, and said, "Are you going to do my biopsy or not?"

It was at that moment that I realized that not everyone wants to help themselves. Not everyone wants to participate in their health, to take control of it. Some people just want the knife, or the pill, or the drug, or the procedure. They don't want to do the work. They don't want the responsibility. For many, it's just easier to blame the system for the failure of their health. I get it. At the same time, I realized that's not who I wanted to partner with. The physician-patient relationship is a partnership. I wanted to partner with people who wanted to be well, believed they could be well, and were willing to do what it took to be well.

I resigned from my surgical position that day.

The health of our society is steadily declining. If the last few years have taught us anything, it's that we are the least healthy we have ever been. Less than 10% of Americans are metabolically healthy. That means that 86% of Americans are walking around with some form of chronic disease, be it being overweight, obesity, hypertension, silent cardiac disease, lung disease, liver disease, diabetes, kidney disease, autoimmune disease, or cancer. These numbers are astounding. And how do we approach this in the medical field? The exact same way we approach acute disease. We treat the symptoms. But unlike the fracture that can be healed by setting the bone or the appendicitis that can be cured by removing the appendix, the acute care model does not work for chronic disease. Are we keeping people alive longer with these methods? Maybe. Are they living better? Definitely not.

Nowhere is this more obvious than in the case of breast cancer. When someone is first diagnosed with breast cancer they turn to their doctor for answers. As a breast cancer surgeon, I was faced with this situation thousands of times. The first question that every single person diagnosed with breast cancer asks is, "Why did this happen?"

My medical training taught me to say that breast cancer is "multifactorial." I would say, "There are several things that contribute to a breast cancer diagnosis over one's lifetime, none of which are within your control."

I would call it "the perfect storm." It is the prevailing opinion of the current medical establishment that breast cancer is just something that happens to people. And while this absolves people of guilt, it is a very damaging mindset. What it ultimately does is rob people of the power that they possess to control their health and their destiny.

By believing that cancer is just something that happens, we abandon our opportunity to see cancer for what it really is. Breast cancer is a normal response to an abnormal environment. People who get breast cancer don't have a bad breast. In fact, there is nothing inherently wrong with the breast. The imbalance is in the system in general. The reason breast cancer develops is because the system failed due to toxic overload, not the breast.

The breast is nothing more than the canary in the coal mine.

It's interesting. The vast majority of my conversations with a potential new patient start like this, "I am healthy except I have breast cancer."

This is a troubling but completely understandable mindset, because most people don't know what it means to be healthy. We think of health as the absence of disease, but that is not entirely accurate. Health is optimal function. As we just learned, there are only about 10% of Americans who are functioning optimally. There is a huge disconnect between what people generally believe is healthy and what being healthy actually is. Traditionally-trained doctors do not understand health. They are only taught to recognize disease. They are taught to recognize when systems fail. However, they do not recognize when health is diminishing. They do not know when and how to redirect people toward health. I myself wasn't able to make the distinction until I got sick. It wasn't until I discovered functional medicine that I was able to see health through a different lens. Because while in the case of breast cancer all the focus is on the tumor, I know that the tumor is not the problem. The tumor is the symptom of the problem. By removing the tumor, radiating the patient, and giving chemotherapy or anti-hormonal therapy, we are not doing anything to positively impact the health of that individual going forward. We are not positively impacting the trajectory of their life. It's much the opposite. The way that we are addressing breast cancer only diminishes health and longevity. While I understand that there are situations in which this conventional approach is necessary, I now know that it is not the solution, and certainly not the answer for most people. However, the functional medicine approach which looks at root cause, which looks to discover the imbalances in the system and correct them, which asks why you got sick, which looks to lower and limit inflammation, and ultimately create an environment that fosters health, this is the answer for everyone. And it's for everyone looking for answers that I wrote this book.

In studying functional medicine, I realized my role as a surgeon in breast cancer patients' journey was useless. While I did beautiful work removing tumors and reshaping breasts, functional medicine taught me that removing the tumor doesn't change anything. Removing the tumor has no impact on what is driving breast cancer and therefore has no impact on whether or not the cancer will return. Adding on radiation or chemotherapy also doesn't address the underlying cause. Therefore, there is nothing to stop the tumor from returning. Even if the cancer doesn't return, as most of them don't, by not addressing the root cause people just go on to manifest the next illness. This approach, this symptom-directed care, is nothing more than a never-ending game of whack-a-mole. You cut off one thing and something else pops up. You give a drug for that and another symptom manifests and on and on it goes. So, intent to get out of this broken system and make a true impact for women suffering under the weight of a breast cancer diagnosis, I left my surgical practice in 2019 and opened Real Health MD to help women to truly heal. I was determined to help women with a breast cancer diagnosis create health and change the trajectory of their lives using functional medicine and its principles. I needed to change the treatment paradigm, to change the way we approached breast cancer. I didn't want to be part of the problem anymore; I wanted to be part of the solution.

Here is how the conventional medical environment really has it wrong. Conventional thinking is that the tumor is some foreign object that is not a part of you. We proclaim war against it. We believe that something is wrong with those rogue cells and that something is wrong with the breast. But the truth is that cancer is a part of you. It's the part of you that is telling you that things aren't working. It's the part of you that doesn't feel safe. Breast cancer is a normal adaptation to an abnormal environment. We'll go into more detail on what breast cancer is in the next chapter, but for now take this away: focusing on the tumor is not the answer, because the cancer itself is not the problem. The problem is the environment. The problem is the host. It sounds unkind, I know, but. . . the problem is you.

You are also the solution.

The Problem with Genetics

Let's talk about genetics for a minute. Breast cancer is so often thought to be a genetic disease. However, only five to ten percent of cancers have a true genetic disposition. Even in those cases, those with BRCA mutations, or PALB-2, or CHEK2, even with those mutations in the cancer suppressor genes, the environment is still of the utmost importance. Genes may load the gun but the environment pulls the trigger. In families where multiple people get breast cancer but there's no known genetic link found, there may be a genetic component, but remember these people also grew up in the same environment. They tend to have similar exposures, similar health and eating habits, and similar dietary and lifestyle habits. Therefore, they are going to experience similar health, or lack thereof. I was trained to believe that the risk factors for breast cancer were age and gender, and that is true. However, I was also made to believe that genetic and family history played a far bigger role than it actually does. The truth is that what causes breast cancer is chronic inflammation. It's chronic inflammation that leads to stress chemistry, which leads to this abnormal cancerous environment. Cancer is an environmental disease. Functional medicine focuses on the environment. It asks, "What's in your environment that's hurting you?" or, "What's not in your environment that you need?"

Inflammation is the New Smoking

Now let's talk about inflammation. Inflammation as a term and a concept is highly misunderstood. Inflammation is neither good nor bad. We need inflammation. It allows us to heal when we cut ourselves, prevents us from dying from the common cold or a bug bite, or from bleeding out when we cut ourselves. Our inflammatory system allows us to recover from a trauma or surgery. Without inflammation, we could never mend a broken leg or survive an accident. Our inflammatory system is a vitally important aspect of our physiology. We need inflammation. However, it's when we're getting constantly bombarded by inflammatory triggers daily from things and places where we shouldn't be getting it, that it builds up and leads to these disease states.

I can't remember a single breast cancer patient in the last twenty years who can't recall some major stressor a year or two preceding her diagnosis. We must remember that we are modern beings living on a very old gene code. That gene code hasn't changed in thousands of years. We are not designed for prolonged periods of inflammation. When coming out of the cave in the morning and encountering a saber tooth tiger, we were either meant to run as quickly as we could and escape the tiger or get eaten. What we are not designed for is to run from the tiger for three days, three weeks, three months, or even three years. We are designed for these quick periods of acute stress followed by long periods of relaxation and relief. Yet many of us live in this constant state of stress or sympathetic overdrive. The saber tooth tigers in our lives are the pressures of daily living: stressful jobs, deadlines, financial worries, difficult relationships, emails, social media, poor sleep, toxins, the pressures of public life, living under a microscope, and a seemingly constant need to do it all. All of this translates to inflammation. Chronic inflammation leads to autoimmune disorders and cardiovascular disease, metabolic disorders like diabetes and fatty liver, bone and joint diseases like osteoarthritis and rheumatoid arthritis, pulmonary diseases like asthma and COPD, neurologic diseases, Alzheimer's and Parkinson's disease, dementia, MS, depression, anxiety, and . . . CANCER. Chronic stress suppresses our immune system. Think about it. Our bodies only know two states: fight or flight or rest and relax. If you are constantly fighting, why would you need to worry about dying from the common cold? When we are in sympathetic overdrive, our immune system is essentially shut off. So, the real reason that we get breast cancer isn't our genes, or bad luck. It's that we have chronic inflammation that builds up over time, exceeding our body's ability to process it, which leads to stress chemistry. We are literally toxic. When in this toxic state, our immune system is turned off. It is the perfect combination for breast cancer. That is "the perfect storm" of breast cancer.

Because the conventional medical system doesn't address the root cause, isn't looking at why people are toxic, and isn't working to restore the health of the immune system, this is why people after breast cancer treatment are far worse off than they were before. This is why people have recurrences, or worse. Removing the cancer, giving chemotherapy, or radiation, or any other drug does not address the underlying inflammation. It doesn't address why someone got sick—why they got cancer. This is why we need functional medicine. What functional medicine looks to do is identify where the inflammation is coming from and mitigate it. More importantly, functional medicine seeks to help you build an anti-inflammatory environment. It helps you create the chemistry of joy, and get rid of the chemistry of stress. Please know that I am not disparaging conventional medicine or physicians. Conventional medicine is filled with many well-intentioned people doing exactly what they were trained to do. In fact, I do not believe in throwing the baby out with the bathwater. There is still a time and a place for traditional cancer treatments. For people with a large tumor burden, they are in need of a quick way to decrease that burden. Their proverbial sink is overflowing. Surgery, chemo, and radiation are ways to mop up the floor. However, the far more important thing is to ultimately figure out how to shut off the faucet. Functional medicine shuts off the faucet. That's what anti-inflammatory living does. Unless you do that, your sink is just going to overflow. I don't tell people not to have surgery, or chemotherapy or radiation. I meet people where they are and with what they need. I never ask people to make a choice of one or the other. It's never an OR for me. It's an AND.

I recognize that everyone diagnosed with breast cancer gets a treatment plan. That's okay. But what every person who gets breast cancer needs is a HEALTH PLAN. Functional medicine provides that health plan.

Functional medicine is changing the paradigm. By understanding that breast cancer is not the disease but the symptom of the disease, we can approach it entirely differently. We are not fighting disease. We are not fighting anything. We are creating health. Breast cancer is not a chemotherapy deficiency, a radiation deficiency, or a surgery deficiency. Therefore, chemotherapy, or radiation, or surgery never cured anyone, and they never will. The cure is in one place—the cure is in you. The cure is in getting to the root cause, changing your path, and embarking on a new journey. But unless you yourself change, you cannot expect change. In fact, the definition of insanity is doing the same thing again and again and expecting a different outcome. What we want to do is see where the path went wrong, and change your path, so that you are moving in the right direction.

In this book, we are going to cover all the different ways to create the health you are looking for. We will introduce the pillars of health, the foundations of anti-inflammatory living. In this book, we'll cover nutrition, nutrients, nourishment, food, supplements, sleep, movement, mindset, stress management, toxins, relationships and the importance of purpose driven living. We will talk about what to do before, during, and after your breast cancer diagnosis, and how to go from diagnosed to survivor to thriver. This book is intended to show you how to create a loving, nurturing, health-building environment so you both heal from breast cancer and know the best health of your life.

This book is my answer to breast cancer.

CHAPTER TWO - WHAT DO I DO?
(WHY YOU SHOULDN'T PANIC)

"You have breast cancer."

These are the four most frightening words a woman will hear.

Ever.

But they don't have to be. I promise you that breast cancer doesn't have to be a life sentence. I understand it feels like a punishment, something you never wanted. I was right there with you. Even though I didn't have cancer, I understand how being diagnosed with a life-threatening disease rattles you to the core. Like many of you, my doctor flat out told me I would die if I did not do the conventional treatment. At that time, I was in my forties with two young children. All I could think of was that I was going to die and leave my husband alone to raise our boys. Breast cancer is not a blessing. . . But it can be an opportunity—an opportunity to take stock of your life in a way that you wouldn't have otherwise. An opportunity for you to look around you and evaluate through a critical lens what is working and what isn't. It's an opportunity to ask whether you are on the right path, living your purpose, or if you have been hijacked by the business of life and are living on someone else's agenda. This can be your opportunity to do better, to be better. Inside this book are the tools for coping with this diagnosis in a controlled and dignified way, while at the same time taking back the power that you lost with your diagnosis. This book aims to educate you and provide you with everything you need to put this diagnosis behind you and get you on the road to a healthier, more vibrant, centered, and meaningful life.

And this is where you start.

Your Diagnosis is Not an Emergency

I know a breast cancer diagnosis feels like an emergency, but with rare exception, it is not. Before we go any further, I want to talk about those exceptions because if they apply to you, I want to make sure that you get the help you need right now.

1. Inflammatory Breast Cancer

Inflammatory breast cancer is one of the forms of breast cancer that needs semi-urgent attention. Most people have plenty of time to learn about breast cancer and the various treatments, assemble their team, and work with them to formulate the best plan. If you have inflammatory changes in your breast, meaning redness, heat, peau d'orange (skin edema, or "skin of the orange"), with an underlying breast cancer (mass), this is something that needs to be addressed now. Inflammatory breast cancer is a clinical diagnosis, meaning that if you have these changes in your skin, along with a breast cancer diagnosis, you should be treated for inflammatory breast cancer (IBC). You do not need a skin biopsy showing cancer in the skin. These changes alone are diagnostic for this form of the disease, and treatment should not be delayed. This form of breast cancer tends to progress very quickly, so each day matters. Women with inflammatory breast cancer report going from having a normal breast to one month later having a red, swollen, hard breast filled with tumor. If this applies to you, please get yourself to a surgeon who can perform a biopsy to get some information about your tumor that will guide treatment and then to the medical oncologist for treatment. Reading the rest of this book will be highly beneficial to you as the tools described in the remainder of this book will benefit you most.

2. Breast Cancer that Has Caused a Fracture

Another exception is if you have breast cancer that has spread to the bone that has caused a fracture. Metastatic disease alone is not an emergency. Most people that present with metastatic disease have had that disease for a very long time. However, if the metastatic disease has progressed to the point of fracture, it is usually accompanied by a significant amount of pain and suffering. It is nearly impossible to heal while you are suffering. In this instance, urgent radiation to the area of fracture can relieve the pain and stop the progression of disease in that area so that you can start to heal. To heal, it is important that you read the remainder of this book so that you have the tools you need for healing.

3. Brain Metastases

Finally, if you have brain metastases, or breast cancer that has spread to the brain, this needs urgent attention. The brain sits in a fixed space, the skull. When cancer spreads to the brain, it both makes the brain bigger (tumor growth) and is a very inflammatory state so there is considerable swelling involved. Eventually, if the brain gets too large, it will herniate from the skull, cutting off the blood supply to the brain. This is a fatal condition, so we want to avoid this situation at all costs. For this reason, someone with brain metastasis needs urgent attention. Anyone with a breast cancer diagnosis who has a change in personality, cognition, or behavior, should have an urgent evaluation for brain metastasis with a CT or an MRI of the brain. Always remember to premedicate for a CT scan or an MRI with the protocols I have laid out in this book (p 192-193).

While the previously described circumstances seem worrisome, and they are, I have seen people reverse their disease even when diagnosed with what seems like end stage disease. Be positive. Read this book. Take control of your life. Healing can happen. At any age, or any stage, healing can happen.

The Twelve Things You Should Know (Right Now)

If none of those previously mentioned circumstances apply to you, then PLEASE take a breath. It's okay at this point if you even breathe a sigh of relief. Take a pause. Get some perspective. You can handle this. Below are the twelve things that you need to know RIGHT NOW. Nothing else is urgent. It may feel that way—breast cancer certainly feels like an emergency. For most, the emergency is an emotional one. For the majority of women, a breast cancer diagnosis is the worst thing to have consciously happened to you. Many of us, myself included, have suppressed very traumatic times in our lives. But, as we know from Dutch psychiatrist, researcher, author and trauma expert, Dr. Bessel van der Kolk's book, The Body Keeps The Score[3], the body truly does just that. What we don't process, what we don't heal, eventually will manifest physically. We will get to all of that. For now, here is what you need to know: I've got you. Breathe. Read this book. Apply the principles. Healing will happen. This book is all about creating health. Decide now that you are going to get healthy. Know that you can get well. Use this book to put the pieces in place to get you there and keep you there. By following what is outlined in this book, you can get there. I have had the awesome privilege of seeing miracles happen every day. There are exceptions to every rule and for those that can see breast cancer as an

---

[3] Kolk, V. D., & Bessel, A. (2014). The Body Keeps the Score: Brain, Mind, and Body in the Healing of Trauma.

opportunity to recapture your health, you can achieve exceptional health, and be exceptional!

The Twelve Most Important Things Your Doctor Isn't Telling You That You Need To Know Right Now:

1. Take a breath. There is no rush. You have plenty of time to make the right decisions for you. This is not an emergency (exceptions are Inflammatory Breast Cancer, or metastatic breast cancer that has caused a bone fracture, brain changes, or you are in unbearable pain).

2. Decide that you want to live, not only survive, but thrive.

3. Commit to doing great things to improve your health.

4. Start your three-week juice fast while you are collecting your information. You can find a recipe to follow in the back of this book. (Note: If you have already completed treatment and you are reading this book, you can still do the juice fast to jump start healing in the body. This is especially good for someone living with metastatic disease who wants to try to turn things around).

5. Gather opinions from several providers in each area. These can be breast surgeons, medical oncologists, radiation oncologists, reconstructive surgeons, integrative oncologists, functional medicine physicians, naturopaths, holistic dentists, etc. You have several months to do this. Don't rush. Do it right!

6. Build your team. Look for experienced providers you like most that hear you, understand you, respect your opinion, and share your vision.

7. Do your reading and own investigation. Start BEFORE you start any therapy. Do not agree to any treatment unless it feels right for you.

8. Get baseline labs. Look at your metabolic health, immune system, inflammation, liver and kidney function, thyroid function, tumor markers, vitamin and mineral levels, hormone levels, and lipid levels. Functional medicine doctors know how to interpret these. Conventional medical doctors generally do not. See the supplemental suggested initial lab sheet and optimal values.

9. Get a CGM (continuous glucose monitor) and start to follow your blood glucose. A guide to using your CGM is available in my resources guide on page 207.

10. Prioritize sleep, daily joyful movement, and self care.

11. Put any unsupportive or toxic relationships on hold for now.
There is currently no room for toxicity in your world.
12. Tell yourself every day that you are capable of healing.
Believe it. Know it.
Are you ready to begin? Time to get organized!

CHAPTER THREE - WHAT IS BREAST CANCER: UNDERSTANDING YOUR DIAGNOSIS AND YOUR PATHOLOGY REPORT

So what exactly is breast cancer?

In the last chapter, we discussed how breast cancer is a breast cell's normal response to an abnormal environment. The next question is:

What makes the environment abnormal?

All the toxic exposures from the outside world that we then bring inside of our world and inside of our bodies contribute to an abnormal environment. These toxins actually cause our chemistry to shift from the chemistry of joy to the chemistry of stress. This stress, either from physical or emotional elements, puts stress on our system, and changes our chemical composition. Breast cancer occurs when there has been some chemical shift in the body that makes the breast cells feel unsafe. When this happens, the cells go into survival mode where they are constantly reproducing. These transformed cells are merely responding to the environmental shift.

Now this alone will not cause cancer. Cancer is the intersection of these cells shifting into survival mode coupled with a weakened immune system. An intact immune system should be able to recognize these wayward cells in their infancy and destroy them before they reach critical mass and become a "tumor." However, for most people, the thing that led to cancer in the first place is chronic inflammation. That same chronic inflammation has exhausted the immune system, preventing it from responding adequately or appropriately. It is important to understand this concept, as the key to reversing cancer is to create a safe environment that fosters health instead of promoting disease.

It is equally important for you to understand that your tumor is a part of you. It is not your enemy, and you are not at war. You are not preparing for a fight. You are preparing for peace. Restoring the health of your internal environment is crucial to the healing process. Try not to identify with or get caught up in the details of your diagnosis. Most of them are meaningless. Ultimately, the only thing that is important is restoring you to health.

All of the language around breast cancer incites violence. People think they are gearing up for a fight. Well-meaning friends and family encourage you to fight this and refer to you as a warrior. This "War on Cancer" was started in 1971 by Richard Nixon when he signed the National Cancer Act into law. Since then, cancer has been dominated by violent language.

But violence is the last thing that someone with cancer needs. In fact, it is the result of a prolonged sympathetic state (or a prolonged stressed state), that allowed the cancer to develop in the first place. Remember: one of the elements necessary for cancer to develop is for the immune system to be compromised. Remember: we are modern beings living on a very old gene code. We only know two states: danger and safety. In danger, we are in survival mode. We are chemically dominated by cortisol, our stress hormone. While in this state there is no need for your body to worry about the common cold. Therefore, one of the actions of cortisol is to turn off the immune system—it is an immunosuppressant. It served us very well during times when we had very limited exposure to danger. Back then, once the danger had passed, we returned to the parasympathetic or safety state. In the safety state, our immune systems were strong and we were in a state of healing.

Modern day life, unfortunately, is filled with danger. While we may not literally be surrounded by saber tooth tigers, our system is not able to distinguish between real or perceived threats. Therefore, we end up steeped in cortisol, our immune systems are shut off, and our health suffers.

Here are the things that we know cause the cell damage that we are talking about and hinder our immune system from functioning correctly and efficiently.

Causes of Breast Cancer
- Chronic inflammation from diet
- Processed foods
- Sedentary lifestyle
- Over-exercise
- Radiation exposure (repeated mammograms, x rays, radiation in childhood, etc.)
- Chronic diseases (obesity, diabetes, thyroid, celiac, inflammatory bowel disease, MS)
- Chronic infections (viral, fungal, mold, Lyme, parasites, bacteria)
- Heavy metals (drinking water, dental amalgams, food, cosmetics)
- Chemical exposures (plastics, pesticides, herbicides, fungicides, preservatives)
- Chronic antibiotic use
- Chronic dental infections or cavitations (everyone with a history of dental work should see a holistic dentist[4])
- Frequent toxin exposure (alcohol, smoking)
- Chronic constipation
- Insomnia
- Chronic sleep deprivation, short sleepers
- Night shift work
- Being overweight
- The Electromagnetic Field (EMFs)
- Unresolved trauma

---

[4] You can find a holistic dentist at https://iaomt.org/.

- Chronic stress from a difficult relationship, bad marriage, or horrible boss
- Being a caregiver to a sick parent, spouse, partner, or child
- Divorce
- Job loss or unwanted move

It is important to remember that breast cancer is not caused by one thing. It is the combination of things that cause cellular damage and immune suppression that culminates in a breast cancer diagnosis. Remember, just like these cells can be transformed into cancer cells, the body can also heal and these processes can be reversed.

Understanding Your Pathology Report

If you have come this far in the book, you probably have a breast cancer diagnosis. That also means that you probably have a pathology report. In my seventeen years as a surgeon, I was often asked to give a second opinion. What I found was most people did not understand their pathology report at all. Most of the time there was minimal effort put toward helping people to understand their diagnosis, and far more effort put toward giving people treatment options. I don't know about you, but I like to understand why I'm going to do something before I do it. Therefore, the following section is here to help you understand your pathology report. I do, however, want you to know this: you are not your tumor, nor are you your pathology report. This is one aspect of what's happening inside of you and in no way represents the totality of what's happening with you. The pathology report describes your tumor (or the small part of your tumor that was sampled, anyway). It describes characteristics of your tumor, like the (size, nodal status, and prognostics like hormonal or HER2 status. Just because your tumor has estrogen receptors on it doesn't mean that you have a problem with estrogen. This is conventional medicine's way of putting you in a bucket so that they can make generalized treatment recommendations. It is crazy to assume that everyone with similar pathology has the same disease and would respond to the same treatment. We are all unique. We all arrived at this diagnosis for different reasons. I wrote this book to help you move forward on the correct path for you. In the words of Emil Faber, President of Faber College, "Knowledge is Good."

The following pages contain a guide for understanding your pathology report.

What are the types of breast cancer?

Your pathology report probably gave your breast cancer a name. Breast cancer is a complex disease, and there are several phenotypic types of breast cancer, each with distinct characteristics under the microscope and behaviors. Breast cancers are named by the normal tissues they most resemble. Invasive ductal carcinomas are characterized by the formation of abnormal ducts. Invasive lobular carcinomas are made up of linear collections of cancer cells growing in a single plane. Here are the main histologic types of breast cancer you will find on your pathology report:

1. Invasive Ductal Carcinoma (IDC): IDC is the most common type of invasive breast cancer, accounting for about 80% of cases. It originates in the milk ducts but then invades the surrounding breast tissue. Invasive cancer cells have the ability to spread beyond the breast. When they grow outside of the ducts into the surrounding tissue, they can access the blood vessels and the lymphatics and travel to other areas of the body through those systems.

2. Invasive Lobular Carcinoma (ILC): ILC begins in the milk-producing glands (lobules) of the breast and then invades nearby breast tissue. It accounts for about 10%-15% of invasive breast cancers. It spreads through the same mechanism as ductal cancers.

3. Invasive Mammary Carcinoma (IMC): IMC has both ductal and lobular characteristics.

4. Inflammatory Breast Cancer (IBC): IBC is a rare and aggressive form of breast cancer. It often presents with redness, swelling, warmth, and a thickened appearance of the breast skin. By definition, inflammatory breast cancer is a breast cancer with overlying inflammatory skin changes (thickening, redness, dimpling (peau d'orange) and other inflammatory changes in the skin of the breast. Unlike other breast cancers, it may not present as a distinct lump. This type of breast cancer is the only one that requires prompt treatment. If you have been diagnosed with inflammatory breast cancer, time is of the essence. This is one of the true breast cancer emergencies.

5. Triple-Negative Breast Cancer (TNBC): TNBC is a subtype of invasive breast cancer that lacks estrogen receptors (ER), progesterone receptors (PR), and does not over-express HER2. It is typically more aggressive and has less treatment options but can respond very well to an integrative approach.

6. Hormone Receptor-Positive Breast Cancer: This type of breast cancer can be of either ductal or lobular origin. It is defined by the presence of estrogen receptors (ER-positive), progesterone receptors (PR-positive), or both ER and PR receptors on the cancer cells. It accounts for most breast cancer cases, and this type of cancer most resembles normal breast tissue which also has Estrogen and Progesterone receptors.

7. HER2-Positive Breast Cancer: HER2-positive breast cancer overexpresses the HER2 protein on the cell surface. Normal breast cells have 20,000 HER2 receptors on their surface. However, there are some breast cancers that overexpress HER2 and have 40 to100 times more HER2 receptors on their surface. We refer to these cancers as HER2-positive. HER2-positive tumors tend to grow faster and can therefore be more aggressive if untreated. Targeted therapies, such as trastuzumab (Herceptin), Pertuzumab, Lapatinib, and Afatinib are effective in targeting the HER2-positive cells and treating this type of breast cancer. Breast cells aren't the only cells to have HER2 receptors. HER2 is also found on many organs including the heart, the skin, the gastrointestinal tract, the respiratory system, the reproductive system, and the urinary system. Treatments aimed at the HER2 receptor will affect all the cells with a HER2 receptor.

8. Metastatic Breast Cancer: Though this is a stage more than a subtype, I think there is an important concept to understand. Metastatic breast cancer, also known as stage IV breast cancer, occurs when a cancer which started in the breast spreads to other organs of the body, such as the bones, liver, skin, lungs, or brain. It is the most advanced stage of breast cancer. There are very rare times when we find breast cancer in other parts of the body but not in the breast. This scenario is not common but it does happen. The important thing to understand here is that if you have breast cancer that has spread to the bones, you do not have bone cancer. You have metastatic breast cancer.

9. Tubular Carcinoma and Mucinous Carcinoma or Colloid Carcinoma: Though rare, these special types have a very favorable prognosis and require very little, if any, treatment beyond surgery.

10. Phyllodes Tumor: Phyllodes tumors are rare sarcomatous cancers of the connective tissue of the breast. Unlike what we generally refer to as breast cancer, which arises from the glandular tissue of the breast, phyllodes tumors arise from the fibrous tissues of the breast. They account for less than 1% of breast tumors. They can be benign, borderline, or malignant. Malignant phyllodes tumors respond mostly to surgery and repeated excisions may be required. Malignant phyllodes tumors can be very aggressive and recur quickly. When they spread, they tend to spread either directly (by growing through the breast into the chest wall, ribs, and eventually lung) or they access the bloodstream and spread that way (we call it hematogenous spread). Fortunately, these types of tumors are very uncommon.

11. Male Breast Cancer: Although rare, breast cancer can also occur in men, representing less than 1% of all breast cancer cases. Male breast cancer is treated the same as female breast cancer. Because men have less breast tissue, and less breast cancer awareness, when they do develop breast cancer they tend to present at later stages.

12. Metaplastic Breast Cancer: Metaplastic breast cancer is a rare and aggressive subtype, representing less than 1% of breast cancers. The tumor cells resemble both glandular (ductal) and non-glandular (sarcomatoid) tissues. These cells tend to be primitive in their appearance. They are fast growing cells that don't often respond to conventional treatments.

13. Paget's Disease of the Breast: Paget's disease of the breast is a rare form of breast cancer that starts in the nipple and areola area. It is recognized by crusting, weeping, painful lesions on the nipple and areola, the pigmented part of the breast. It accounts for about 1-4% of cases. It is a non-invasive cancer when found alone but it can be seen in conjunction with an underlying invasive cancer of the breast.

As you can see, breast cancer is a highly diverse disease, and individual cases may exhibit various combinations of these types, making each person's disease and treatment plan unique. This is also why no two people will respond to conventional treatment in the same way, AND why conventional treatments do not universally work. Everyone's disease is different because everyone's why is different. The type of cancer you have is less important than recognizing that there is a why: there is an imbalance in the system that needs to be corrected. Because breast cancer is not a chemotherapy deficiency, or a radiation deficiency, those modalities will not restore balance (Though they may be necessary at times, for a short amount of time, for instance with advanced or aggressive disease).

I encourage you to use this book to help you to recognize how to figure out your why and create a healing environment. If you give your body what it needs to heal and remove the things that trigger illness, health happens.

What About the Things That Aren't Breast Cancer?

The road to breast cancer is neither predictable nor linear. This means that we don't know that something that is precancerous is then going to be cancerous and then metastatic. In fact, there is evidence to the contrary. The vast majority of women diagnosed with Ductal Carcinoma In Situ (DCIS) never go on to develop outright breast cancer or invasive disease. There are several lesions seen on mammogram, or biopsy, some of which are spoken about as if they are precancerous, or worse yet, you are told they are cancer. Many times, when these cell types are seen on biopsies, people are made to think that even if it is not cancer now, it is most certainly going to be. This may be true for those of you who do nothing to live your life differently tomorrow than you did yesterday. But, if you bought this book, you already suspect there is something more—something that you're not finding in the conventional medical system. You are at least thinking about change, if not already committed to it. In the following pages, I discuss some cell types that, in my opinion, should do nothing but prompt change in you. Remember, anything that is not cancer is benign and should be thought of and considered that way. In fact, a National Cancer Institute working group in 2013 recommended that the name "carcinoma" be removed from DCIS to highlight the fact that the lesions aren't quite malignant, and therefore may not need the more aggressive treatment that cancers would warrant. The American Association for Cancer Research (AACR) states, "Around twenty percent of DCIS cases eventually transform into invasive cancer or recur after the primary tumor is removed."[5]

That means that 80% won't progress and do not need treatment of any kind. Also, this data is based on the assumption that people undergo conventional treatment and do not modify their disease-causing risk factors at all. That is not you. You are here because you want to do more, learn more, and be better. If you have any of these findings, it should be looked at as a blessing more than anything else. You do not have cancer. You are presented with the opportunity to change. Your body is giving you a warning, sending you a signal. These are the whispers. Listen to the message from your body, and you can prevent the screams. Use this as an opportunity to give your body what it needs.

Cell Types That Are Not Cancer
1. Ductal Carcinoma In Situ (DCIS): DCIS is a non-invasive breast lesion that occupies the milk ducts. It is most often diagnosed on a biopsy following the discovery of calcifications on a mammogram. Calcifications occur due to some underlying process, in this case DCIS. It is important to remember that calcium itself is not the problem. The

---

[5]Jones, Calley, PhD. 2022. "Ductal Carcinoma in Situ: The Weight of the Word 'Cancer' - American Association for Cancer Research (AACR)." American Association for Cancer Research (AACR). October 13, 2022.

problem is the underlying inflammatory change that is happening on the cellular level. In Situ means the process has not spread beyond the ducts into the surrounding breast tissue. DCIS, because it is contained within the ductal system, has no potential to metastasize or spread. In order for a cancer to spread from the breast to other areas of the body, it would do so in one of two ways: by blood or through lymphatics. These structures are located OUTSIDE of the ductal system in the breast. Therefore, DCIS has no access to the bloodstream or the lymphatic system. This is why it has no potential to spread or be life threatening. Anyone can live without a breast. I am in no way suggesting that you have your breast removed. I say this solely for your understanding that DCIS is not a threat to life. For this reason, it is highly debatable as to whether this should be considered cancer, or even precancerous. In my practice, I view it as a call to action. At the same time, I think it is important to note that women who get treated for DCIS have a shortened lifespan. They are not, however, dying of breast cancer. They are dying of heart disease—heart disease that is accelerated by "treating" the DCIS. This, my friends, is a huge problem. More about this later. Another important point here is that if you are diagnosed with DCIS, your goal is not to reverse the calcifications, your goal is to reverse the inflammation.

2. Lobular Carcinoma In Situ (LCIS): LCIS represents an expansion of the cells that make up the breast lobules (the milk producing units of the breast). Unlike lobular cancer (ILC), this is a non-invasive lesion. In fact, most people would hesitate to even call it a lesion. Much of the time, LCIS is discovered incidentally on a breast biopsy performed for something else. When we see LCIS on a biopsy, we consider that a risk factor, meaning that you have an increased likelihood of developing breast cancer in the future. However, this by no means implies that you are destined for breast cancer. In fact, if you use this opportunity to employ the modalities discussed in this book, you can mitigate that risk and turn this process around. The name, LCIS, like it's cousin DCIS, is unfortunate, alarming, and frankly inappropriate.

3. Atypical Ductal Hyperplasia (ADH): ADH represents an overgrowth of cells within the duct. A normal duct when seen in a cross section contains one layer of cells. However, if there is an inflammatory process happening within the duct, then these cells start to overgrow and heap up atop one another. If they do this in an orderly fashion, we call it Usual Ductal Hyperplasia. However, if the cells start to mutate, a transformative process that cancer cells undergo, and they start to arrange themselves in an irregular way, then we call that Atypical Ductal Hyperplasia, or ADH. ADH can exist on its own or be on the periphery of breast cancer. The finding on a biopsy of ADH does slightly increase your chance of getting a subsequent breast cancer, however only if you do nothing differently going forward. That is not you!

4. Atypical Lobular Hyperplasia (ALH): Like its cousin ADH, ALH is noted when the cells within the breast lobules expand in number. These cells typically look and behave differently than normal lobular cells but don't meet the criteria for LCIS.

What Stage Am I?

Beyond a diagnosis, the first question people ask me is, "What stage am I?" Even though people have no idea what that means, they are intent on getting that information. The problem is, they then get the stage and the grade confused because the terminology and the way they are reported are similar. I want to take this time to explain the reporting systems to you so that you know the difference, you understand your report, and then you file that information away because it means virtually nothing. It is an archaic system that does little to predict treatment or long-term outcome today.

What is the TNM System for Breast Cancer?

Our breast cancer staging is based on both anatomic, and since 2017, prognostic factors. The anatomic system is the TNM staging system. It stands for Tumor, Node, and Metastasis. In 2017, we started to include the status of the following biomarkers: human epidermal growth factor receptor 2 (HER2), estrogen receptor (ER), and progesterone receptor

(PR). This staging system, based on a stage of 0 through IV, is used to make five year survival predictions. Since five years is a nominal amount of time, this attempt at staging is largely meaningless. However, it is still universally practiced so I included it here. Here's how the TNM staging system works:

Tumor (T)

- **TX:** Tumor size cannot be assessed
- **T0:** No evidence of tumor
- **Tis:** Carcinoma in situ (abnormal cells are present but are contained within the duct)
- **T1:** Tumor is 2 cm or less in diameter
- **T2:** Tumor is more than 2 cm but not more than 5 cm in diameter
- **T3:** Tumor is more than 5 cm in diameter
- **T4:** Tumor has invaded the muscles of the chest wall (pectoralis muscles) or the skin

Node (N):

- **NX:** Lymph nodes cannot be assessed
- **N0:** No lymph node involvement
- **N1:** Cancer has spread to one to three axillary (armpit) lymph nodes, or to the internal mammary nodes (located beneath the breast by the sternum or chest bone)
- **N2:** Cancer has spread to four to nine axillary lymph nodes or to the ipsilateral (same side) internal mammary nodes
- **N3:** Cancer has spread to ten or more axillary lymph nodes, or to the infraclavicular (located beneath the collarbone) or supraclavicular (located above the collarbone) lymph nodes

Metastasis (M):

- **MX:** Presence of metastasis cannot be assessed

- **M0**: No evidence of distant metastasis
- **M1**: Cancer has spread to distant organs such as the lungs, liver, skin, brain, or bones. It is important to note that if a breast tumor breaks directly through the skin, this is considered direct extension, or T4, but not metastatic (stage IV).

The combination of T, N, and M stages determine the overall stage of breast cancer, ranging from stage 0 to stage IV. This staging system helps conventional doctors determine their treatment plan based on the amount of tumor burden. It is also used as a way of predicting five-year survival of breast cancer.[6]

What are breast cancer grades? What do they mean?

Breast cancer is graded based on how abnormal the cancer cells look under a microscope. Essentially, pathologists look to determine how much or how little they resemble normal breast tissue. They also are looking for growth rate. The less the cells resemble normal breast cells, the higher the grade. The more cells that are in mitosis (the process of dividing or replicating), the higher the grade.

Here are the three grades of breast cancer:
- **Grade 1 (low grade):** The cancer cells look most like normal breast cells and have very few if any cells in mitosis.
- **Grade 2 (intermediate grade):** The cancer cells look somewhat abnormal and are reproducing at a moderate rate.
- **Grade 3 (high grade):** The cancer cells look very abnormal and are reproducing quickly.

[6] Iwai, Tomohiro, Masao Yoshida, Hiroyuki Ono, Naomi Kakushima, Kohei Takizawa, Masaki Tanaka, Noboru Kawata, et al. 2017. "Natural History of Early Gastric Cancer: A Case Report and Literature Review." Daehan Wiam Haghoeji 17 (1): 88. https://doi.org/10.5230/jgc.2017.17.e9.

The grade of breast cancer is one of the factors used in determining which treatments are appropriate for you. Grade 1 breast cancer is typically less aggressive and does not respond to chemotherapy, while Grade 3 breast cancers are more aggressive and may benefit from more aggressive modalities. Your oncologist will consider the cancer grade along with other factors, such as the stage and biology, to determine the most appropriate treatment plan for you.

What are the breast cancer stages?

Breast cancer is typically classified into five stages, which are determined by the size and spread of the tumor. These are the five stages of breast cancer:

Stage 0: This is also called ductal carcinoma in situ (DCIS), which means the abnormal cells are confined to the milk ducts (it has not grown outside of the ductal system). This is meaningful because without leaving the ducts, it has no potential to get into the bloodstream or the lymphatic system. These are the ways in which breast cancer spreads (metastasizes). Because DCIS has no potential to spread, it is 100% curable. No one dies of DCIS. The decision as to whether to treat DCIS is debatable. As DCIS is not cancer, strong consideration should be given to health optimization instead of treatment at this stage. Everyone will say that they know someone who died of DCIS. That is not true. Because breast cancers are heterogeneous, that means that not all of the tumor is the same. There can be times when the breast lesion contains both DCIS and invasive disease. We typically only sample a portion of any lesion. Therefore, there are instances, although rare, when we believe there is no invasive cancer when there actually is. Our current system is very imperfect. Cancers are missed all the time. However, if you have a diagnosis of DCIS you should trust in the fact that you are in no rush to treat. This is especially true if the lesion is small and if there is no mass (lump) involved. Instead, I recommend you do all you can to maximize your health.

Stage 1: At this stage, the tumor is small (less than two centimeters), is contained to that breast, and has not spread to the lymph nodes on that side. Stage I breast cancers are almost universally curable. However, there will be a small percentage of women with stage I disease, by virtue of the tumor being small and not present in the lymph nodes, that have aggressive biology. Aggressive biology is aggressive biology and though these women are technically stage I, they do not have predictable outcomes. Women with aggressive disease, even when found early, can have poor outcomes. With our current system, it is hard to identify these women. However, liquid biopsies with genetic analysis do a far better job of analyzing the tumors and predicting their behavior compared to our current staging system.

Stage 2: The tumor is larger (between two and five centimeters) and/or has spread to nearby lymph nodes.

Stage 3: The tumor is larger (greater than five centimeters) and has spread to nearby lymph nodes, or has invaded nearby tissues, such as the chest wall or skin. Tumors that reach this stage typically have more aggressive biology and behavior.

Stage 4: This is also known as metastatic breast cancer, where cancer has spread to distant organs such as the lungs, liver, brain, or bones.

I again want to stress that using grade, size, and nodal information alone to stage cancer and predict outcome is outdated. Now that we have a greater understanding of tumor behavior and have biologic information to predict outcomes, this old staging system is unreliable. Please remember that this staging system is just a crude and imperfect way of predicting survival. I would pay far less attention to the stage and more attention to what might be causing your breast cancer.

Will I Survive This?

The next question I am asked following, "What is my stage?" is, "Am I going to live?" I understand this question. I asked the very same question myself in 2017. The truth? We are all going to die eventually. However, it shouldn't be now and it shouldn't be from breast cancer. It also shouldn't be in five years, however that is what the current staging system predicts: five-year survival. In the scheme of things, for most of us, five years is NOTHING! I don't know about you, but I don't want to know about five years. I want to know,

"Am I going to live a long life?"

The average American woman lives to eighty-three, and I am not average! I don't want you to be average either. That said, as you go on your breast cancer journey you are going to encounter many doctors who are going to give you lots of statistics. This is what they are referring to: the five-year survival of breast cancer according to stage.

PUTTING IT ALL TOGETHER: To view the clinical prognostic stage table, visit: https://emedicine.medscape.com/article/2007112-overview.

What Are The Five-Year Survival Rates for Breast Cancer Patients? The five-year survival rate is the percentage of people who survive at least five years after being diagnosed with breast cancer. The survival rate for breast cancer varies based on several factors, including the stage of the cancer at diagnosis. Here are the estimated five-year survival rates for breast cancer by stage:

- **Stage 0:** DCIS—close to 100%
- **Stage I:** about 99%
- **Stage II:** about 93%
- **Stage III:** about 72%
- **Stage IV:** about 27%

It's important to remember that these are estimated survival rates based on large groups of people and do not take into account individual factors such as age, overall health, comorbidities (which in the case of breast cancer there are often many) and specific characteristics of the cancer.

I again want to point out that I think to talk about a five-year survival in the context of breast cancer is a ridiculous amount of time. The vast majority of breast cancers are very slow growing, and a five-year time period does not truly reflect survival. Surviving five years is not survival.

What You Should Know About Your Tumor Cells

Breast cancer cells develop from normal breast cells. As such, many of them resemble normal breast cells. The more they resemble normal breast cells, the more they behave like normal breast cells, the better the prognosis. Here are some of the tumor characteristics that we look for both for diagnostic and treatment purposes:

Tumor size: The size of the tumor is one factor used in determining the stage of breast cancer and planning appropriate treatment strategies.

Histologic grade: Histologic grade assesses the appearance of cancer cells under a microscope and helps determine how different the cancer cells are from normal breast cells. A higher-grade tumor means it looks less like a normal cell and is associated with more aggressive behavior and faster growth.

Hormone receptor status: Hormone receptors, including estrogen receptor (ER) and progesterone receptor (PR), indicate whether the cancer cells have receptors on their surface for estrogen and progesterone. It is important to know that normal breast cells have estrogen and progesterone receptors on them. Hormone positive tumors are made up of cancer cells that have an increased number of hormone receptors on their cell surface compared to a normal breast cell. This does not, in any way, mean that hormones cause breast cancer. This is association but not a causation. Increased numbers of the hormone receptors on a cancer cell is that cell's survival adaptation. It is totally unrelated to having too much hormone. Hormone receptor-positive tumors are often treated with medicine that targets the estrogen receptor. We do not target the progesterone receptor because we don't currently have drugs to do that (and because the side effects of that drug would be practically intolerable).

HER2 Status: Human epidermal growth factor receptor 2 (HER2) is a normal protein found on the surface of breast cells. In some breast cancers, that HER2 protein can be over-expressed, meaning that there are too many of them. We call these HER2+ tumors. HER2-positive tumors may respond to targeted therapies specifically designed to affect HER2-positive cells. It is important to note that there are normal cells in the body that have the HER2 protein on their surface, like cardiac (heart), gut, respiratory, reproductive, and genitourinary cells. Therefore, any treatment that targets HER2-positive cells will also target the heart and other organs, potentially causing damage to these normal vital organs.

Ki-67 Index: Ki-67 is a protein associated with cell proliferation. A higher Ki-67 index suggests faster tumor growth due to rapid cell division and potential for more aggressive tumor behavior.

Presence of ductal carcinoma in situ (DCIS): DCIS is a non-invasive breast condition that is defined by an overgrowth of abnormal cells within the duct. This condition is confined to the milk ducts. Its presence in addition to an invasive lesion may influence treatment decisions, and lead to larger resections and more aggressive treatment in an attempt to "get it all."

Other Molecular Markers

Additional molecular markers and genomic features can provide further insights into the tumor's behavior and potential response to treatment. Before agreeing to any treatment, you should make sure with your medical oncologist that you and the tumor have had full biologic and genetic analysis. You want to ensure that whatever treatment plan you are given is personal and going to be effective for you, as most are not. There are tests used to predict response to chemotherapy and hormonal therapy, like the Oncotype, the MammaPrint, the Breast Cancer Index, and others. Remember that these tests only predict likelihood of recurrence and then assume those with a high likelihood of recurrence would be the only ones to benefit from chemotherapy or extended hormonal therapy. These tests do not predict your individual likelihood of response to therapy. They are merely a predictor of who should consider systemic therapy like chemotherapy or extended hormone blockade, and who should not.

There are genomic tests that can be run on your tumor to determine your response to certain drugs. Again, while these tests identify mutations of your tumor, they do not predict your response to the corresponding drug. Many integrative oncologists choose to take the testing further. There are tests like the RGCC or DATAR that can predict INDIVIDUAL response to therapy. This kind of individual testing is not commonly done within the conventional medical system as it is generally not covered by insurance, and, more importantly, requires a considerable amount of individual time and attention. Cancer treatment currently is based on standard protocols and is not geared toward individualized care. The time for change is now. (More on this later.)

Now that you have the basics, the remainder of this book is going to provide you with a roadmap to determine the best path forward for you. It will help you to decide who you work with and what you need to do to put your breast cancer diagnosis behind you.

Remember, the findings in your pathology report are only describing a small part of you—the tumor. YOU ARE NOT YOUR BREAST CANCER so try not to identify as such. You are not hormone positive, triple negative, or HER2 positive. The characteristics of your breast tumor, along with your overall health, medical history, and preferences, are used by your team to develop your personalized treatment plan. The ultimate goal is to tailor treatment to your unique circumstances, maximizing the likelihood of a successful outcome and minimizing potential side effects—both in the short and long term. Remember that the vast majority of women survive breast cancer. As such, we want to ensure that you are neither under-treated nor over-treated. If you are to survive breast cancer, which you more than likely will, you should have a life worth living. The thing you need to prepare most for is LIVING. That is what this book is all about!

CHAPTER FOUR - HOW IS BREAST CANCER "TREATED"?

Conventional breast cancer treatment recommendations depend on several factors, including the size of the tumor, the stage and extent of the cancer, tumor biology, your overall health, and personal preferences. Remember that these treatments are solely aimed at the tumor and will do nothing to correct why the breast cancer is there. That is up to you. Helping to figure out your why is on the subsequent pages of this book.

Here are the standard treatment options:

Surgery: Surgery is often the first treatment recommended for breast cancer and involves removing the cancerous tissue from the breast. The type of surgery depends on the size and location of the tumor and may include lumpectomy (removal of the tumor and some surrounding tissue) or mastectomy (removal of the entire breast). At the time of surgery, if you are being treated for an invasive cancer, the neighboring lymph nodes underneath the arm are often sampled and removed. If you are being treated for DCIS with lumpectomy, there is no role for lymph node sampling.

Cryoablation: Cryoablation is an emerging technique in the treatment of breast cancer. This involves freezing the tumor and some surrounding tissue. Its application is currently being limited to those with small, early-stage tumors under 1.5 cm in diameter. There also must be little to no DCIS, as extensive DCIS makes the tumor margin less predictable. There are ongoing studies as to who is the ideal candidate for this treatment. I am confident that this minimally invasive therapy will be proven effective and become popularized by women who are looking for less invasive ways to treat breast cancer.

Radiation therapy: Radiation therapy uses high-energy radiation to kill cancer cells and reduce the risk of cancer recurrence. It may be used after surgery to destroy any remaining cancer cells. Recent evidence suggests that radiation may no longer be routinely necessary as it DOES NOT impact survival.

Chemotherapy: Chemotherapy involves the use of powerful drugs to kill cancer cells throughout the body. It may be used before surgery to shrink the tumor allowing you to be a candidate for lumpectomy if you aren't already, or after surgery to kill any remaining circulating cancer cells. Chemotherapy is not a selective treatment. It is delivered into your bloodstream and travels throughout your body. It kills both cancer cells and normal cells.

Hormone therapy: Hormone therapy is used to block the effects of hormones that may stimulate the growth of certain types of breast cancer. It is used in combination with other treatments or on its own. Note that all of our current hormonal treatments involve manipulation of estrogen or the estrogen receptor. However, numerous studies have shown estrogen to be protective against breast cancer and breast cancer recurrence.[7]

Targeted therapy: Targeted therapy involves the use of drugs that target specific proteins or genes that may contribute to the growth of cancer cells. An example of this includes Herceptin (Trastuzumab) directed against the HER2-positive cell. This can be given alone or in combination with chemotherapy. Note that when Trastuzumab is given along with chemotherapy, there are far greater side effects and damage to normal tissues.

---

[7]Manyonda, Isaac, Vikram Talaulikar, Roxanna Pirhadi, John H. Ward, Dibyesh Banerjee, and Joseph Onwude. 2022. "Could Perimenopausal Estrogen Prevent Breast Cancer? Exploring the Differential Effects of Estrogen-Only Versus Combined Hormone Replacement Therapy." Journal of Clinical Medicine Research 14 (1): 1–7. https://doi.org/10.14740/jocmr4646.

Off label therapy or repurposed drugs: There are many pharmaceuticals approved for other purposes that have anti-cancer activity. We will explore some of these drugs later on in this book. However, for a full discussion on the use of off label drugs to reverse cancer, I recommend that you read How To Starve Cancer by Jane McLelland.

Nutrients and Supplements: There are many nutrients and supplements that can help to both reverse cancer and recover your health. We'll discuss these later in this book.

Assembling Your Team

Your recommended treatment plan for breast cancer will vary depending on your individual characteristics. Your team of healthcare providers, including a surgeon, medical oncologist, radiation oncologist, integrative oncologist, naturopath, and functional medicine provider will work together to develop a personalized treatment plan aimed at addressing your cancer. Please remember that the tumor is not the problem. The tumor is the symptom of the problem. You should be working twice as hard at improving your health as you are at targeting the tumor. The goal of your team should be to protect you and promote your health above all else.

Before agreeing to any treatment plan, it is important to assemble your team. On your team, you are going to want to have:

- A Breast Surgeon
- A Medical Oncologist
- A Radiation Oncologist
- An Integrative Oncologist
- A Functional Medicine Physician or Naturopathic Doctor
- A Cancer Coach
- Supportive friends and family

It would be nice if all of these individuals worked cooperatively with one another. I believe that is what the future has in store for us.

Unfortunately, we are still operating in a very fragmented system where each practitioner only knows and takes responsibility for their part. Very few conventional practitioners think globally or holistically. That is why it is so important to have integrative practitioners on your team.

How to Build Your Team

1. Medical Team Members: When choosing your medical team, it is important to work with people who instill a sense of calm, of trust, availability and concern for larger implications. The big picture is important. The vast majority of people will survive their breast cancer diagnosis. Your quality of life after treatment is of the utmost importance. You want to work with someone who recognizes that. It is also important to work with someone who is respectful of your beliefs and allows for your opinions to be heard. It is important for your medical and radiation oncologist to know that your goal is health and not just completing treatment. (Over-treating is probably the biggest problem people encounter with medical and radiation oncologists today.) Someone who listens to you and is more concerned with your health and wellbeing than the protocol is the person that you want to work with. If you are working with an integrative oncologist already, great! If you are working with conventional oncologists, make sure they are aware of, or at least open to, integrative measures to improve outcomes. Integrative oncologists recognize that there is a time and a place for chemotherapy but that standard regimens are inappropriate. They are finding innovative and proven ways to deliver less chemotherapy with better outcomes. Instead of offering standard doses of chemotherapy, most integrative oncologists suggest low dose continuous chemotherapy or metronomic chemotherapy. In addition, they are taking advantage of the hyper-metabolic characteristic of cancer cells and using insulin potentiation therapy. This involves administering insulin at the same time as chemotherapy drugs, with the idea that lower chemotherapy doses are then needed because insulin lets more of the drug enter cells. This is done in combination with fasting so that the normal cells are protected from chemotherapy exposure. While there is good evidence that these methods are superior in terms of patient tolerance, response, and outcomes, they are not being readily adopted by conventional cancer treatment centers. This is why it is important to explore including an integrative oncologist on your team and take an active role in your plan.

2. Personal Team Members: Identify what your needs are and assign them to the best person for the job. Diversification is key. Acknowledge people's strengths and their willingness and excitement to help. Be willing to accept help as it will enrich your journey. Just be reasonable and insightful about assigning tasks to people. Don't give a friend who hates to cook the job of making dinners. Don't ask your busiest friend to bring you to your appointments. Play to people's strengths and know that they want to help. Allow them to. Teamwork makes the dream work!

3. Community: Identify your people and make spending time with them a priority. These people should bring you comfort and joy. At the same time, you should not include the people that don't agree with you or are telling you what you should do, especially when what they want doesn't align with what you want. The only opinion that matters right now is yours. You want to surround yourself with YES'S! right now. Put the naysayers and the negative nellies on hold for later.

4. Volunteer: You may feel as if you don't have much to give right now, but I can tell you that there is always someone less fortunate than you. There is always someone who knows less, has less, or has done less. People can always benefit from your experience and what you learned. Helping others is one of the best ways to heal.

5. Create Purpose: Living with purpose is the best way to ensure longevity. Allowing your diagnosis to redefine your purpose is a way to create something positive out of your experience.

Now that you have assembled your team, and identified potential partners on your healing journey, it is time to get down to business. I have assembled all the questions you need to ask your providers in the following chapters and in a downloadable PDF in my resources guide on page 207.

CHAPTER FIVE - WHAT SHOULD I ASK MY DOCTOR?

I find that most people get a diagnosis, go to a doctor, and have no idea what questions to ask. I wrote this book partially to prepare you thoroughly for that exact situation. This chapter is broken up by sections according to specialty. It contains the questions you should be asking, along with the supportive information you will need in order to understand the answers. These materials will guide you toward making the right decisions for you.

In case you wanted to print these questions out, they are also available in my resources guide on page 207.

Questions for your Functional Medicine Doctor or Naturopath

If you're lucky, you will have access to an integrative oncologist in your area to help support you and bridge the gap between conventional cancer care and functional medicine. However, because integrative cancer care is still not commonplace, many of you will only have access to people that practice functional medicine without necessarily specializing in cancer. There are great advantages in having a functional medicine provider on your team, even if they don't specifically specialize in breast cancer.

Here are some questions to ask to make sure you and your provider are a fit for one another and that you feel that it would be beneficial to work together on your health. Everyone with breast cancer gets a treatment plan. However, the one thing that everyone with breast cancer really needs is a health plan. A functional medicine provider can help you to create that health plan.

- How familiar are you with treating breast cancer patients?
- What are the advantages of using functional medicine to address breast cancer?
- Can you share some examples of women like me who you have successfully worked with?
- What is your approach?
- How would you go about creating a health plan for me?
- What kind of testing do you do?
- What is the purpose of functional testing?
- How do you use the information you get from the testing?
- How do you tailor treatment plans to individual patients?
- What will be required of me as your patient?
- What kind of diet do you recommend?
- What lifestyle modifications, such as stress reduction techniques or exercise, do you suggest in support of my health?
- How will we track my progress?
- How frequently will I need to undergo tests and assessments?
- Will you interpret the results of these tests and adjust my treatment plan accordingly?
- How do you collaborate with my oncologist or other medical specialists involved in my care?
- Do you provide guidance on potential interactions between functional medicine treatments and conventional cancer therapies?
- Will you counsel me when making both functional and conventional treatment decisions?
- What are the potential risks and benefits associated with the functional medicine treatments you're recommending?
- Will you help me to determine what caused my cancer?
- How does functional medicine contribute to my long-term health and prevent recurrence?
- What are the long-term strategies for reducing the risk of breast cancer recurrence?

- What steps can I take to support my immune system and overall well-being?
- Can you provide scientific research or studies that support the use of functional medicine for breast cancer patients?
- Are there specific treatments that you recommend? (High dose Vitamin C? Mistletoe? Ozone? Low Dose Naltrexone (LDN))? How do you determine who benefits from these therapies? Do you provide these therapies?
- How do you stay updated on the latest developments and research in functional medicine? What about Breast Cancer?
- What is the estimated cost of working with you and over what period of time?
- Will my health insurance cover any of the cost?
- Do you have a support team? Health coaches? What will their role be in my care?
- Are you open to my working with other functional medicine practitioners or conventional oncologists?
- Do you see people in person or virtually?
- Is there anyone you won't work with, and why?
- Do you have patient testimonials that you can share with me?
- Do I need to see a biologic dentist? (Hint: the answer here should always be yes.)

The functional medicine approach is vastly different from the conventional medical approach. Unlike conventional medicine, which is completely focused on the tumor, functional medicine doctors realize that the tumor is not the problem. The tumor is the symptom of the problem. Therefore, what functional medicine looks to do is to get to the root cause of whatever is driving your disease.

I am unique in that I was a cancer doctor before a functional medicine doctor. As such, I am as comfortable with cancer as I am with functional medicine. It is unlikely that you will find someone with a background just like mine. That does not mean that you can't find a wonderful provider to help you. Just be sure that the person you choose to work with is comfortable with cancer. You need that. In the end, the functional approach is similar no matter what background you come from: By eliminating whatever drives illness, you can create health.

This is done by establishing the pillars of wellness. These pillars include your diet, fasting, prioritizing movement and sleep, finding productive ways to cope with stress, avoiding toxins, beginning detoxification, releasing trauma, and living a connected, purpose-driven life. We'll cover all of these pillars later in this book; for now, know that functional medical doctors, even the ones that are not accustomed to dealing with cancer, are accustomed to digging deep, getting to the root cause of inflammation, and helping you to identify what is interfering with your health and establishing equilibrium.

Functional medical doctors know that our bodies are one system playing in concert. You can not have a symphony unless everything is working together in harmony. A functional medical doctor can help you to establish harmony.

To learn more and be a part of my functional medicine community, join https://www.facebook.com/groups/keepingabreastwdrjenn/.

Questions to Ask Your Breast Surgeon

The breast surgeon is usually the first doctor you will consult with after receiving a breast cancer diagnosis. Sometimes, they are the ones that did your biopsy and gave you the diagnosis. After receiving your diagnosis, your breast surgeon will usually evaluate the extent of your disease, explain your diagnosis to you, talk to you about your general state of health, arrange for testing, give you a clinical stage, and then present you with treatment options after putting all of that information together. Your surgical options will depend on:

- The size of your tumor in relation to your breast size.
- Whether there is one or multiple tumors.
- Whether or not you desire to keep your breast.
- Whether or not you have local or systemic (metastatic) disease.
- What the goals of surgery are (curative versus palliative ie. decreasing the tumor burden).

When making your decision, an important fact to keep in mind is that the likelihood of survival is exactly the same whether you decide to keep your breast or remove it. Having counseled thousands of women through this decision, here are my words of wisdom: If you have your breast removed, no matter how good the reconstruction, there will never come a day from that day forward where you won't remember that you had breast cancer. However, if you choose to keep your breast, and your surgeon does a good job with your surgery, there will come a time where you are no longer defined by your breast cancer. In my experience, removing your breast no matter how prepared you think you are for it will leave deep scars, far beyond what you see in your skin. You may not always have a choice, but when you do I recommend breast conservation surgery or even better, cryoablation. Cryoablation is a minimally invasive technique done under ultrasound guidance that involves freezing the tumor.

Here are the questions you should be discussing with your breast surgeon while making your treatment plan.

What are the different surgical options available for me?

Understand the various surgical procedures that may be suitable for your specific breast cancer. These may be:
- Cryoablation
- Lumpectomy or breast conserving surgery
- Mastectomy or complete removal of the breast
- Partial or complete reconstructive options

What is the recommended surgical approach for my case, and why?

Ask your surgeon to explain why a particular surgical option is being recommended, considering factors like the size of your breast cancer in relation to your breast size, where the tumor is located, whether it is a single tumor or multiple, your overall health, personal preferences, and what is important to you.

Do I need lymph node sampling?

With invasive cancers, it is customary to sample the lymph nodes. The lymph node status is then used to help predict likelihood of metastasis and benefit from systemic therapies like chemo. If you have a small tumor (less than 5 mm), a sentinel lymph node biopsy is unnecessary unless the tumor has extremely aggressive biology or the lymph nodes are clinically suspicious. A clinically suspicious lymph node is enlarged and can be felt on a physical exam or seen on ultrasound. The most common lymph node procedure performed today is called a sentinel lymph node biopsy.

If you are having a sentinel lymph node biopsy, ask the surgeon to explain how they do the procedure to you.

Ask how they locate the sentinel node, whether they use blue dye, radioactive tracer, or both. Ask if they do preoperative imaging of the node. If they do imaging or use radioactive tracers, this would be additional radiation, so you should take 100 mg of melatonin and 2,000-4,000 mg of liposomal Vitamin C the morning of surgery with a sip of water.

Also, ask if they have patients with lymphedema from a sentinel lymph node biopsy and what can be done to prevent it.
They should have an answer for you. It should involve early mobilization, daily range of motion exercises, and weight training from here on out.

If you have known lymph node disease, an axillary dissection will likely be suggested.
Ask to have that procedure explained to you and ask about their incidence of complications with that procedure. Known complications of ANY axillary surgery are:
- Numbness of the skin
- Decreased range of motion of that arm (early mobility, daily range of motion exercises, and weight training all help to prevent decreased range of motion)
- Lymphedema, or swelling of the arm (also prevented by early mobility, range of motion exercises and weight training)
- Winging of the scapula comes from damage to the long thoracic nerve during surgery. This is a concern for anyone undergoing axillary surgery or total mastectomy, but is a rare complication

Will my nipple(s) be affected?
Ask about nipple involvement, whether it will be altered or removed, and whether the nipple will have sensation and function afterward.

Will you be placing semi permanent markers in to guide you for the surgery?
Will they come out at the time of surgery? Note, some of these markers are radioactive so be sure to inquire about your doctor's technique.

Will you be putting semi permanent or permanent markers in my breast at the time of surgery?

What will you use and what are the risks of having permanent markers in my breast? Most of the time titanium clips are placed in the surgical bed at the time of lumpectomy. In my practice, I used Biosorb which is a biodegradable space occupying scaffold that also contains tiny titanium wires to mark the previous tumor cavity while preventing deformity.

How will the surgery affect my breast's appearance and sensation?

Ask what you can expect your breast to look like after the surgery. Where will your incision be? Will you be symmetrical? Will you keep your nipple? Will you have sensation? If you are interested in changing the breast at the time of your surgery (i.e., having a breast reduction or lift), ask if there is a plastic surgeon that they work with who can be present at the time of your surgery to improve the cosmetic outcome of the procedure. Typically, when a plastic surgeon is involved, they will perform a symmetry procedure and make the non-cancerous side match the cancerous side if that is important to you.

If you are undergoing mastectomy, ask if it will be skin sparing and/or nipple sparing.

Oftentimes, it is possible to retain the skin and nipples with mastectomy, creating a very natural appearance in the reconstructed breast. It is important to note that this breast may look natural, but it will not be functional.

If I am to have a mastectomy with reconstruction, what kind of reconstruction would you recommend?

Would it be immediate at the time of my mastectomy, or delayed? Is there a reconstructive surgeon that you work with that you recommend?

Would you let the reconstructive surgeon you recommend operate on your family member?

Am I a candidate for cryoablation?

Cryoablation is a minimally invasive technique that utilizes very cold temperatures to freeze the tumor. This procedure is done under ultrasound guidance. It is ideal for people with one tumor in the breast that is less than 1.5 cm (about 0.59 in) in diameter. Following this, the tumor is no longer viable and is resorbed by the body. While this technique is still under investigation, the results are very promising. If you have an early-stage single tumor, this may be an option for you. In addition, for those with metastatic disease that wish to decrease their tumor burden without having surgery, this is a viable option.

How long will it take to heal? What are the common complications of this surgery?

What are the potential risks and complications associated with the surgery being proposed?
Make sure you have a comprehensive understanding of the possible risks and complications of the recommended surgery, and how they might be managed before agreeing to and scheduling anything. Anytime anyone undergoes surgery, there is a risk of bleeding and infection. Ask your doctor how to minimize those risks.

What are the expected benefits and outcomes of the surgery?
Discuss the expected outcomes of the surgery, the goal of the surgery (is it curative?), what the breast will look and feel like, and how and when the surgery will fit into the overall treatment plan.

What type of anesthesia will be used during the surgery?
Understand the type of anesthesia planned for the procedure and discuss any concerns you may have. Most of the time, breast conserving surgery alone can be done using sedation and local anesthesia. Mastectomies or surgery on both breasts will usually be done under general anesthesia. Ask about the anesthesia risks as well. Be sure to tell your doctor about any previous problems you have had with anesthesia so that they can come up with a safe plan for you.

What can I expect in terms of post-operative recovery and healing?
Ask about the recovery process, including pain management, wound care, and any restrictions on activities after surgery. Please see the attached document on preparing for breast surgery. Breast surgery is rarely painful. Any discomfort can usually be managed with over-the-counter pain medicines. You want to try to avoid narcotics as they are immune suppressive and increase the likelihood of recurrence. In addition, they are highly constipating and negatively impact your microbiome.

Will I need any additional treatments after surgery, such as radiation or chemotherapy?

Discuss the possibility of additional treatments that may be required after surgery to start to prepare yourself for what your team is thinking.

What are the alternatives to surgery, if any?

Inquire about non-surgical options that might be available for your breast condition and discuss their effectiveness. People are having great success with cryoablation so that is a great option for those that are candidates.

How experienced are you in performing the type of surgery you are recommending for me?

Discuss the surgeon's experience and expertise in breast surgery to ensure you are in capable hands. It is important that you trust your breast surgeon as this is going to be an important relationship for you.

Are there any lifestyle changes or preparations I should make before the surgery?

Inquire about any pre-surgery instructions, such as dietary changes, smoking cessation, alcohol cessation, medications, or supplements to avoid.

If this is a recurrence surgery, and you have had radiation in the past, inquire about doing HBOT prior to and following your surgery to maximize your chances of healing.

The Guide to Breast Surgery (here and available for download in my resources guide on page 207) will give you most of the instructions you need but it is important to review them with your doctor. I recommend reading them over several times so that you can prepare yourself for the best surgical outcome.

Remember, your breast surgeon is an essential part of your healthcare team, and open communication is vital in order to make informed decisions about your breast surgery. Feel free to ask any additional questions that come to mind to ensure you feel comfortable and confident in your chosen treatment path. There is no rush for you to make your decision. Whatever decision you make you will more than likely live with for a very long time so it is important to make the right one for YOU!

Questions to Ask Your Medical Oncologist

Chemotherapy is a systemic treatment used to decrease the amount of tumor burden, shrink tumors, or prevent them from returning. It is generally recommended when there is significant tumor burden, or when the lymph nodes contain tumor, or in the event of aggressive biology. Before agreeing to chemotherapy treatment for breast cancer, it's essential to have a clear understanding of the therapy and its potential impact on your health and well-being both during and after treatment. I recommend pursuing integrative oncology for the best possible outcome. Integrative oncology is about combining the best of conventional, integrative, and complementary approaches to support your health and well-being during breast cancer treatment and beyond. Modern chemotherapeutic regimens should be highly individual, and recommendations should be based on thorough biologic and genetic analysis of the tumor. In addition, everyone with breast cancer should be undergoing genetic testing to see if there are therapeutic and preventative measures available specifically to them.

Here are the most important questions to ask your medical oncologist BEFORE deciding whether to include chemotherapy into your personalized plan.

- **What is the specific type and stage of my breast cancer?** Understanding the type and stage of breast cancer will help you grasp the rationale behind the recommended chemotherapy treatment and its potential benefits. In general, only late-stage cancers or cancers with aggressive biology benefit from chemotherapy.
- **What is my risk of recurrence?**
- **What tests were used to determine that risk and which factors influenced that risk?**
- **Has my cancer been fully tested for all the latest biologic and genetic markers that can be used for targeted care?** Make sure that your tumor has been tested beyond ER, PR, HER-2, Ki-67, and other basic markers. We now have biologic targets that can be tested for which have targeted therapies. Ask the medical oncologist which tests were done.
- **What are the goals of chemotherapy in my case?** Determine whether chemotherapy is intended to shrink tumors before surgery (neoadjuvant therapy), treat remaining

58

cancer cells after surgery (adjuvant therapy), or control the cancer if it has become metastatic (palliative therapy).

• **Which chemotherapeutic drugs treatments are recommended for my cancer, and why?** Understand the specific drug treatments, why they are being recommended to you, and their potential benefits for your breast cancer type and stage. Be sure to ask about the percentage of people who typically benefit from the drug and what their impact is on SURVIVAL. You are not interested in any other surrogate endpoints. Tumor shrinkage alone has not been associated with long term survival. If the drug is being recommended to extend life, ask how long the average person benefits from the drug. Many of these drugs only extend life by a few weeks and are very difficult to tolerate. Be sure to inquire what characteristics of your tumor make you a good candidate for the treatment being recommended. We are in the age of individualized cancer care. Any treatment recommended should be specific to the biologic and genetic makeup of you and your tumor.

• **Are you willing to consider and prescribe off label drugs known to have therapeutic effects in treating cancer?** Certain pharmaceutical drugs, like statins, NSAIDS, certain antibiotics, anti-parasitics, and antihistamines have been found to have anti-cancer effects when used for short periods of time during treatment. Please read How To Starve Cancer by Jane McLelland for more information.

• **What are the potential risks and benefits of chemotherapy for my condition?** Discuss the expected outcomes of chemotherapy in your case, including improvements in survival rates and reducing the risk of cancer recurrence. Be sure that you are getting absolute survival rates and not relative. Understanding the potential side effects will help you prepare for the treatment and decide if the benefits outweigh the risks in your situation. Most chemotherapeutic drugs have long term consequences including but not limited to heart damage, disturbance to the microbiome, acceleration of heart disease, weight gain, immunosuppression, hair, nail and skin damage, nerve damage, and brain inflammation leading to brain fog and difficulty with memory, computing, and recall. For what is often minimal benefit, you want to be sure that you are not trading one problem for several larger ones.

• **Are there integrative therapies that can complement conventional treatment?** Inquire about integrative therapies, such as acupuncture, mind-body techniques, nutritional support, exercise, fasting, nutrients or herbal supplements, that may enhance your quality of life during and after treatment. Specifically, your doctor should know or understand the benefits of fasting before and during chemotherapy treatments and how certain supplements, like high dose IV Vitamin C, ozone, and HBOT enhance the efficacy of chemotherapy while protecting your normal cells.

• **How might integrative therapies help manage treatment side effects?** Discuss how integrative therapies like fasting can help reduce side effects like nausea, fatigue, pain, depression, anxiety, and immunosuppression associated with conventional chemotherapy treatments.

• **Are there any specific potential interactions between integrative therapies and conventional treatments or medications that concern you?** It's crucial to ensure that any complementary therapies you consider will not interfere with the effectiveness of your prescribed treatments. At the same time, you want to know that you are doing the most to benefit yourself while undergoing treatment, which often requires the use of integrative therapies.

• **Are you okay with my working with an integrative oncologist or complementary cancer therapy specialist?** If you are interested in an integrative, holistic approach, and your current oncologist is not familiar with integrative therapies, ask if they can refer you to a specialist who can provide guidance and recommendations. If they do not know of anyone, make sure they are comfortable working alongside the integrative practitioner you identify. If they are not open to cooperative care, and that is what you are looking for, this may not be the right oncologist for you.

• **Are there specific lifestyle changes or dietary modifications that could benefit my treatment outcomes?** Discuss the role of diet, exercise, stress management, fasting, supplementation, and other lifestyle factors in supporting your overall health and response to treatment. If your doctor doesn't believe these are important, this may not be the ideal person for you to work with.

• **How will chemotherapy affect my daily life?** Understand the potential impact of chemotherapy on your ability to work, exercise, travel, or engage in regular activities, and discuss strategies for managing any disruptions.

• **Are there clinical trials available for my type of breast cancer?** Inquire about ongoing clinical trials that may offer access to innovative and less harmful treatments and potentially improve outcomes.

• **What is the long-term outlook after chemotherapy?** Discuss the prognosis after completing chemotherapy, including follow-up care and monitoring for any signs of cancer recurrence. Make sure the absolute benefits of chemotherapy are presented to you.

• **What would happen if I were to refuse chemotherapy and instead make dietary and lifestyle changes to improve my health? How much benefit does adding chemotherapy actually add?** Remember, you want absolute benefit and not relative.

• **If I optimize my weight, adopt an anti-inflammatory diet, exercise daily, manage my stress, reduce my toxic load, and improve my overall health, do I still need chemotherapy? How much will chemo benefit me?** An honest medical oncologist will say, "I don't know." If they say it will not benefit you and that you need chemo, I would be wary of that practitioner as one of your partners.

Remember to take notes during the conversation with your oncologist or bring a trusted friend or family member with you to help remember important details. It's crucial to have an open and honest discussion with your medical oncologist to make well-informed decisions about your breast cancer treatment. It is also important that your doctor understands that you want an integrative approach. They should respect your perspective and desire to be an active participant in your care. Should you decide to include chemotherapy in your treatment plan, remember to practice the fasting mimicking diet before and during your chemotherapy treatments. You can learn more about this in the fasting section.

Ultimately, breast cancer is not a chemotherapy deficiency, and chemotherapy won't cure you. The only person who can heal you is YOU!

Other Questions to Consider

Is Tamoxifen Right for Me? Tamoxifen is commonly prescribed to premenopausal women with estrogen receptor-positive breast cancer. Before taking tamoxifen, it is important to understand what it is, what it does, how it works, and whether it would be a worthwhile addition to your treatment plan.

The first thing you need to understand is that estrogen DOES NOT cause breast cancer. God would not give you a hormone in your body that is so vital to life that causes cancer. That simplistic theory was created by the pharmaceutical industry to sell you synthetic estrogens, like tamoxifen. Breast cells are supposed to have estrogen and progesterone receptors on them. Estrogen receptors on cancer cells do not make them abnormal. In fact, the breast cancers that lack estrogen and progesterone receptors are more abnormal, more aggressive, and more difficult to treat.

Tamoxifen is a synthetic estrogen. It occupies the estrogen receptors on the breast cells. In the breast, like estrogen, tamoxifen is protective against breast cancer. Because it is a synthetic estrogen, it can act on other estrogen receptors around the body, like the uterus. However, unlike in the breast, tamoxifen in the uterus is stimulatory. Women who take tamoxifen have an increased risk of developing uterine cancer, which is why tamoxifen is classified as a known carcinogen. Other common side effects of tamoxifen include hot flashes, nausea and vomiting, fatigue, menstrual changes, vaginal dryness or discharge, mood changes, bone and joint pain, and an increased risk of blood clots.

The efficacy of tamoxifen will vary from person to person. This is because tamoxifen is a pro drug. Tamoxifen must be converted in the liver by enzymes CYP3A4 and CYP2D6 to endoxifen, the active form of the drug. People with slow CPY3A4 and CYP2D6 enzymes do not convert tamoxifen well and do not get much benefit from the drug. You can test these enzymes to see if you are a tamoxifen metabolizer or not.

There are natural alternatives to tamoxifen. It is important to remember that the best thing you can do after being diagnosed with a hormone positive breast cancer are:
- Optimize your weight.

- Eat a phytonutrient rich diet that includes phyto (plant) estrogens like soy, flax, red clover, chickpeas, sesame seeds, tempeh, mung beans and pumpkin seeds.
- Move your body several times a day, especially after eating.
- Build, or at least maintain, muscle mass.
- Prioritize sleep.
- Manage stress.
- Avoid toxins, especially environmental estrogens (plastics, phthalates, fragrance, flavors, antibiotics, sanitizers, etc.).
- Have daily detoxification practices.
- Live a meaningful, connected, purposeful life.

Before deciding on tamoxifen or any other treatment, it's important to discuss your medical history, current health status, potential side effects, and other available treatment options with your healthcare provider. They can provide you with personalized advice based on your specific situation and help you make an informed decision that is best for your health and well-being. Tamoxifen is not suitable for everyone and its risks and benefits should first be carefully assessed. I recommend you read Estrogen Matters by Avrum Bluming and Carol Tavris before committing to taking Tamoxifen.

Should I Take an Aromatase Inhibitor? Aromatase Inhibitors, or AIs, are commonly prescribed to postmenopausal women with estrogen-positive breast cancer. They are believed to work by reducing the body's production of estrogen. AIs are only prescribed to women who no longer have functioning ovaries, so the amount of circulating estrogen is already negligible. We do not use these medicines in premenopausal women with functioning ovaries and significant estrogen levels, as the AIs don't affect ovarian production of estrogen. Before taking an AI, it is important to understand what they are, how they work, what they do, and whether they would be of significant benefit to you. There are long term implications to taking AIs, so it is important to be aware of them before making your decision.

When considering taking an AI, discuss the potential benefit of taking them. Ask what your risk of recurrence is and how much taking an AI will decrease that risk. Ask for absolute and not relative numbers as the absolute numbers will be far less impressive. Make sure the side effects of taking an aromatase inhibitor are well explained. They include:
- Joint and muscle pain

- Hot flashes
- Fatigue
- Bone loss
- Vaginal dryness and discomfort
- Urinary incontinence: Be sure to discuss this with your doctor and ask if you are a candidate for vaginal estrogen (Spoiler alert: you are.)
- Mood changes
- Depression
- Anxiety
- Brain fog
- Sleep disturbance
- Increased cholesterol levels
- Increased risk of cardiovascular events
- Increased risk of Osteoporosis-related fractures
- Loss of libido
- Hair loss and thinning
- Dry skin and hair

Recent reports have found that women treated for breast cancer are two to three times more likely to die of heart disease than women that didn't have breast cancer. This is in part due to the unresolved inflammation that caused breast cancer in the first place, but the other reason is that the treatments for breast cancer, including radiation, chemotherapy, and aromatase inhibitors, all accelerate heart disease. Women in every decade of their life beyond the age of thirty die exponentially more from heart disease than breast cancer. Prior to deciding whether an aromatase inhibitor would benefit you, have your heart health assessed with a CT calcium score (be sure to use the radiation protection protocol in the back of the book). In addition, understand what estrogen withdrawal would mean to your overall health by reading Estrogen Matters by Avrum Bluming and Carol Tavris.

An additional factor to consider is the effect of an AI on bone health. The number of women that die every year following a fracture is the same as those that die of breast cancer. Taking a drug that increases your fracture risk may be trading in one problem for another. There are many natural aromatase inhibitors and incorporating them in your daily diet would give you all the benefits without the harmful side effects. See the Daily Eight Guide in the back of the book to plan what you should be eating moving forward.

Questions to ask Your Radiation Oncologist

When you are considering radiation therapy, it's essential to have an open, honest, and informative discussion with the radiation oncologist. You first need to understand the treatment modality in general, and then decide if it is something that adds benefit to your individual case. Radiation involves delivery of X-rays to the area where the cancer was (or is) with the intention of killing any remaining cancer cells. Unfortunately, radiation is not a selective treatment and does damage normal tissues. Radiation DOES NOT increase survival. You need to know and understand that BEFORE going for your consultation. As it does not contribute to cure, it is important for you to understand the potential benefits as there are significant side effects involved. Radiation is a carcinogen itself, meaning that it causes cancer, so you would need a worthwhile reason to assume that risk.

Here are some of the most important questions for you to ask to determine if you would benefit from radiation:

- **What are the benefits of radiation for my specific breast cancer case?** Understand why radiation therapy is being recommended for your particular breast cancer type, stage, and other individual factors. Ask: What are the specific reasons for recommending radiation for me?
- **What type of radiation plan do you think would benefit me?** Radiation treatment plans vary according to the type of cancer you had, the surgical treatment you chose, and the extent and location of your disease. If the disease was limited to one quadrant of the breast, partial breast radiation might be an option for you. This involves a shorter duration of therapy directed solely at the area where the tumor was. The goal here would be to prevent tumor recurrence. If the tumor was more extensive, or there was lymph node involvement, your doctor will likely recommend whole breast radiation. In some instances, like painful metastases of the bone, or places where the disease is inoperable, like the lung or the brain, radiation is sometimes used as a localized treatment.
- **What are the goals or intentions of radiation therapy in my treatment plan?** To be clear, radiation does not affect survival. Radiation only decreases the likelihood of local recurrence (disease in the breast). Discuss the intentions for

65

radiation therapy for you. Is it to decrease the likelihood of cancer coming back in the breast? Is it because you had a positive sentinel lymph node biopsy without an axillary dissection (removal of the remainder of the nodes). Is it intended to alleviate pain? Is it to control the cancer's growth and symptoms if it has spread and other treatment alternatives have failed?

• **What are the possible side effects and risks of radiation therapy?**Gain a comprehensive understanding of the potential short-term and long-term side effects. In the short term, radiation is known to cause fatigue, redness, skin changes, swelling, blistering, and burning of the skin. In the long term, radiation is associated with fibrosis (hardening of the breast), shrinkage of the breast, lymphedema or swelling of the breast and arm, hyperpigmentation of the skin of the breast (sometimes permanent), loss of elasticity of the muscle of the chest wall, brittle ribs making you vulnerable to rib fractures, thickening and firmness of the muscles of the heart, heart muscle damage, damage to the vessels of the heart increasing the risk of heart disease, damage to the lung, and cancer. These factors must be considered as radiation has adverse effects in nearly 100% of people who undergo it.

• **How will the radiation therapy be administered?** Inquire about your proposed treatment schedule, the number of sessions, and the duration of each session to help plan your daily life during treatment.

• **Will I need to undergo any imaging or simulations before radiation therapy?** Understand the process of simulation and imaging to precisely target the radiation and minimize damage to healthy tissues. Remember to use the radiation protection protocol prior to any radiation emitting imaging or therapy. Discuss the supplements you plan to take with your radiation oncologist and make sure that everyone is on the same page.

　　o You can find the supplements recommended during radiation in my resources guide on page 207.

• **How can I prepare for radiation therapy?** Ask about any pre-treatment preparations, dietary recommendations, and lifestyle changes that may optimize the effectiveness of the therapy. Be sure to ask your radiation oncologist about which supplements need to be discontinued during treatment. Most times, radiation oncologists recommend cessation of all supplements while receiving radiation. Vitamin D, probiotics, magnesium, zinc, melatonin, turmeric, and B-vitamins are all safe to take during radiation (and encouraged). There are also certain supplements that will act as radiation sensitizers and are advantageous to take during radiation. These include turmeric, genistein, resveratrol, reishi mushroom (Ganoderma lucidum) and turkey tail mushroom. I have found that topical melatonin applied to your skin can help to minimize the skin side effects and decrease skin damage. It is important to continue on your whole food, plant-based, grain-free diet plan and maintain your fasting routine during radiation and beyond. Radiation treatments are cumulative so you may not experience any symptoms of radiation in the beginning, but the effects will continue long after you finish your treatments. A diet high in phytonutrients, long fasting windows, and proper supplementation will help your body to combat some of the tissue damage that accompanies radiation and will significantly aid in your recovery.

• **Can I continue working and performing regular activities during radiation treatment?** Discuss the impact of radiation therapy on your daily life, including whether you may need time off work and how to manage any treatment-related fatigue. If you follow the recommendations in this guide, most people will find that they are able to continue to work and be productive during radiation. You should plan for rest and short naps if you need them during radiation treatment.

• **Can I take any medications or supplements during radiation therapy?** Inquire about the use of medications or supplements that may interact with radiation treatment or affect its efficacy. Make sure you discuss these supplements in particular because they are known to be beneficial: turmeric, resveratrol, genistein, reishi, and turkey tail. Ginger, garlic, cinnamon and blueberries in your diet also protect against radiation damage.

• **Are there any complementary therapies that may help manage side effects?** Discuss the potential use of complementary therapies, such as creams for skin irritation or techniques to alleviate fatigue. Exercise during radiation is one of the best ways to combat radiation induced fatigue. Plan to fit your fifteen minute walks in first thing in the morning and then following each meal. Acupuncture is also helpful at alleviating radiation induced fatigue.

• **How will my progress be monitored during radiation therapy?** Ask your radiation oncologist how often you will be seen, what will be checked at each appointment, and how they are tracking your progress. What kinds of things will they be looking for and checking? Will radiation be straight through for the duration, or will there be breaks? What would be the reason for breaks? How do you decide when to resume radiation?

• **What are the long-term concerns after completing radiation therapy and how will they be monitored?**

• **What do I do to recover from radiation?** Ask your doctor about the best ways to recover from radiation. Your recovery plan should include resumption of antioxidants (Vitamins C, E, fish oil, alpha-lipoic acid, melatonin, etc.), your nutrient dense diet with herbs and spices, consumption of lemon balm tea a few times every day for a month, being active every day, and prioritizing sleep.

• **Can I eat foods with antioxidants in them during radiation?** The plant-based diet that is being recommended in this book is full of antioxidants. The amount of antioxidants contained in food will not adversely affect radiation. However, supplementing with antioxidants is not advised while going through treatment. It is important to maintain your nourishing diet while getting radiation.

Remember, radiation is used as an adjunctive therapy in breast cancer treatment. Though it does not increase survival, it can be valuable in pain control, or provide a treatment modality for disease that is not operable. When undergoing radiation, refer to this guide to prepare yourself for the most success with the least damage. When undergoing radiation, open communication with your radiation oncologist is crucial to making informed decisions about your breast cancer treatment. Don't hesitate to ask questions and seek clarification until you have a clear understanding of the treatment plan and the potential benefit of including radiation.

Questions to ask Your Plastic Surgeon

Whether you are having breast conserving surgery or mastectomy, there may be a role for a reconstructive surgeon in your treatment plan. If you are having lumpectomy, you may want to take this opportunity to make your breasts smaller, shapelier, or more symmetrical. If you are having mastectomy, you may want to consider reconstructive options. You may be having one side done and want a symmetry operation on the opposite side. You may be having both breasts done and want reconstructive surgery. When considering breast reconstruction surgery, it's essential to have a detailed discussion with your reconstructive breast surgeon. Here are some important questions to ask:

- **What are the different types of breast reconstruction and which options are available to me?** Understand the various breast reconstruction techniques, such as implants, autologous tissue (rotational or free flap) reconstruction, or a combination of both. What you are offered will depend on the amount of tissue you have, the amount of tissue you need, the health of your tissues, and your general state of health.
- **Which breast reconstruction method do you recommend for my specific case, and why?** Ask your surgeon to explain why a particular breast reconstruction method is being recommended and why. Make sure they are taking into account factors like your anatomy, medical history, and personal preferences.
- **Can you make my breasts symmetrical?** This is especially important if you are having a cancer operation on one side and you want the opposite side to match.
- **What are the potential risks and complications associated with breast reconstruction surgery?** Gain a comprehensive understanding of the possible risks and complications related to the chosen reconstruction method. Every procedure has risks, but some have more than others. Make sure you understand what is involved with the various procedures so that you can make the right decision for you.
- **What will my reconstructed breast(s) look like? Feel like?** Discuss the expected outcome in terms of breast aesthetics, symmetry, and the potential impact on sensation and tissue health.

- **Will the breast reconstruction be performed at the same time as mastectomy or at a later stage?** Discuss the timing of the reconstruction and whether it will be done immediately following your cancer operation or at a future time. If you are considering immediate breast reconstruction, discuss the benefits and drawbacks compared to delayed reconstruction. I always recommend immediate reconstruction whenever possible.
- **How many stages are typically involved in the breast reconstruction process that is being recommended?** Understand the number of surgical stages (procedures and operations) needed to complete your breast reconstruction and the expected timeline.
- **What can I expect in terms of post-operative recovery and healing from breast reconstruction surgery?** Ask about the recovery process, including pain management, wound care, and any restrictions on activities after surgery. Ask about length of hospitalization, drains, dressing changes, need for suture removal, and whether you will need assistance when you go home from the hospital. Ask which activities are permitted and which aren't. Understand when you can return to exercise, lifting, tennis, dancing, swimming, skiing, etc.
- **Are there any potential long-term effects or changes I should be aware of?** Ask about muscle weakness, long term restrictions, loss of function, loss of sensation, need for follow up surgeries, complications of surgeries, and the expected lifespan of the reconstruction.
- **Can I see before-and-after photos of patients who have undergone similar breast reconstruction?** Request to see before-and-after images of other patients who underwent your intended procedure(s) to better understand the final appearance and potential results of the surgery.
- **Will additional procedures be needed to achieve the desired breast appearance, such as nipple reconstruction or revisions?** Discuss any additional procedures that may be required to achieve the final and desired outcome.
- **Can you connect me with people who have undergone this procedure with you before? What are they happy with? What are they unhappy with?**

- **Which reconstruction that I am a candidate for are people the happiest with?**
- **How experienced are you in performing breast reconstruction surgeries?**

Discuss the surgeon's experience and expertise in breast reconstruction to ensure you are in capable hands. If you are planning on having a DIEP flap or other microsurgery, be sure that you are doing that in a center where they do several every week. You want to be sure that your surgeon is very experienced with the reconstruction you choose.

Remember, open communication with your reconstructive breast surgeon is crucial to making an informed decision about your breast reconstruction surgery. Oftentimes, the reconstruction is the most difficult part of surgery and healing from reconstructive surgery takes time and patience. Feel free to ask any additional questions that come to mind ensuring you are fully informed and confident in your chosen path of breast reconstruction.

This team that you're assembling are going to be your partners. In many cases, they are going to provide the conduit to your health. Choose wisely, dial into and trust your instincts. My friend and mentor, Dr. Sachin Patel, says that the patient is the doctor of the future. No one will ever know you better than you know yourself. That is not to say that you are solely responsible-quite the opposite. It means that you are the most important part of this team and you get the deciding vote. It's time to be the CEO of your health. You can do it!

CHAPTER SIX - HOW, WHEN AND WHAT TO EAT

One of the first questions that I get asked from someone diagnosed with breast cancer is, "What should I eat?"

I believe there is a common misconception that there is one best way to eat to either prevent or reverse cancer. I do not believe this to be true. We are all bio-individual and what works best for me may not work best for you, and vice versa. That said, how, when, and what you eat will have profound effects on your health and your outcome. What's right may not be exceedingly clear but what's wrong is.

You're Doing it Wrong

As someone who was a teenager in the '80s, my dietary dogma was born out of the prevailing belief of the time: fat is bad. I was only too happy to accept this fact as gospel. Intent on being thin and thinking the only way to do that was to count calories and avoid "fattening" foods, I traded in my avocado and nuts for breakfast cereal, pasta and Snackwells. After all, they're fat free! I don't have to tell you how that worked out. I spent my senior year in high school and my freshman year in college an easy thirty pounds overweight. My father would say things like, "I know you're the head cheerleader, but you look more like an offensive lineman."

Though his snarky comments were hurtful and wholly uncalled for, he wasn't wrong. Putting it in historical context, he would describe my sister as resembling our French ancestors, thin as a reed, while I represented our Russian heritage. My father would refer to me as "not being afraid of a strong wind." I guess that meant sturdy, and that I was. My weight truly bothered me. Though I have always had what is referred to as an "athletic" figure, I was really pushing the envelope. I tried every fad diet there was. I would lose a few pounds but then binge my way back to being overweight the second I stopped restricting. Then, by complete accident in my sophomore year of college, I stumbled upon what is referred to today as intermittent fasting or time restricted eating. I didn't know it at the time, but fasting was the way in which I would learn to control my weight and my inflammation.

I remember seeing one of my classmates, Tara, coming back from summer break looking thin and fantastic. We were just returning to school sophomore year and it seemed as if a quarter of her was missing. She was thin, her skin was glowing, and she just looked vibrant. The diet junkie in me needed to know what happened. I cornered Tara the moment I could.

"Tara, you look phenomenal. What are you doing?" She said,

"I stopped eating after 6:00 o'clock."

"That's it? There has to be more to it than that."

"Nope," Tara said, "I eat whatever I want to eat during the day but I don't put a morsel of food in my mouth after 6:00 at night."

The early adopter I am started that day. Twenty pounds fell off me in no time. I couldn't have been happier.

This is not a diet book. I use this point to illustrate the fact that weight gain is one of the major indicators of inflammation and carrying extra weight is a major risk factor for the development of and recurrence for breast cancer. To be healthy, we must learn to optimize our weight. This is one of the ways.

When You Eat Matters

You would have to live under a rock to not know about the latest greatest diet trend: fasting. Only, it's not a trend. Fasting has been around since the beginning of time. Every single religion has some sort of fasting built in. Jewish people have four fast days a year, Christians have Lent, Muslims have Ramadan. Our ancestors were wise and understood that in order to be healthy you had to practice some kind of abstinence from food. From an evolutionary standpoint, we are designed to function as well in a fasted state as we are in a fed state. Maybe even better.

Picture this: you come out of the cave in the morning and you encounter a saber- toothed tiger. You haven't eaten yet that day. You turn to said tiger and say, "Can you give me a minute? I haven't had my breakfast yet."

I don't think so.

Our bodies were designed so that even in a fasting state we could run like hell from a tiger. In a fasted state we could hunt and gather, which we did. In a fasted state we could fight wars, cross deserts and oceans, and think with the utmost clarity. We could do just about anything we had to do because food was either abundant or absent and we were designed to acclimate to either situation.

Fast forward thousands of years to the agricultural revolution and better yet, refrigeration. We now have methods of growing and storing food year-round. There are no winters anymore. There is no scarcity. As a result, obesity rates have skyrocketed. Heart disease has risen tremendously. Cancer is at an all-time high. As you will see further along in this chapter and in subsequent chapters, this is one of the major contributors as to why.

The Power of Fasting and Why It Works.

There is research that indicates that fasting can help you both reverse and prevent chronic diseases, like breast cancer, and ultimately live longer.

To understand why fasting is so important, you must first understand what happens when we fast. Fasting turns on our healing mechanisms. Studies suggest that longer fasts, in excess of forty-eight hours, can turn on more healing switches within ourselves which have a multitude of benefits to women. The data out of USC from Valter Longo[8] is quite compelling. Fasting plays a pivotal role not only in preventing disease, but in reversing and treating it.

As humans, we have two main fuels that our cells get their energy from: carbohydrates (sugar) or fat. Starchy carbohydrates (like grains and potatoes) are rapidly converted to sugar or glucose in our bodies. After consuming a carbohydrate rich meal, blood sugar levels increase. As a result, insulin increases, and a cascade of events go into motion, ultimately creating energy for the cells. The problem arises when we consume more sugar than we need. Because we don't store sugar well, we convert what we don't need for fat storage. Excess sugar consumption (and this includes grains, flours made from grains, sugar, syrup, juice, agave, molasses, corn, and whole grains) raises insulin, raises growth factors, and creates a variety of disease states. If you eat too many carbohydrates and store them as fat, it is okay as long as you abstain from food long enough to call on that fat and use it for energy. Problems arise when you eat too much sugar, store what you don't need, and then before you can mobilize it, you have another meal. This is what frequent meals and snacking do. They set you up for weight gain and metabolic disease. In addition, when your body is reliant on glucose for fuel, and because it is not efficiently stored, you have a near constant need for replenishment. However, after about eight hours, or if sugar is not available, your body will switch over to our other energy source—fat. Unlike sugar, fat burning does not increase insulin levels. Instead of causing disease states, it reverses disease states. In general, it takes about eight hours after your last meal for your body to shift to its fat burning system.

The health benefits of using fat for fuel are vast. One of the most comprehensive analyses ever done on the science of fasting was published in the New England Journal of Medicine in December 2019. The authors reviewed more than eighty-five studies and found that intermittent fasting should be used as the first line treatment for obesity, diabetes, cardiovascular disease, neurodegenerative brain conditions, and

[8] Caffa I, Spagnolo V, Vernieri C, et al. 2020. Fasting-mimicking diet and hormone therapy induce breast cancer regression. Nature. https://doi.org/10.1038/s41586-020-2502-7

CANCER. It also stated that intermittent fasting has anti-aging effects and can help with pre and post-surgery healing. This is why I instruct all of my patients to fast an entire twenty-four hours before surgery AND not resume eating until they are hungry. Hunger is the body's signal that it is ready for food.

Despite the overwhelming data in favor of fasting as a vehicle to health, it is not being utilized in the conventional medical system! When was the last time your medical oncologist instructed you to fast? In my experience, you are being told quite the opposite.

By limiting our daily eating window to eight hours or less, and practicing time restricted eating or intermittent fasting, we lower body fat, visceral fat (the dangerous fat that covers the internal organs and sends inflammatory cancer promoting signals into circulation), waist circumference (a marker of metabolic health), blood pressure, LDL cholesterol, and hemoglobin A1C (a three-month marker of blood glucose). Fasting is also associated with a reduction in c-reactive protein (CRP), a sensitive marker of systemic inflammation.[9]

Sandy's Story

Sandy came to see me after she had been diagnosed with a right breast cancer for which she underwent lumpectomy. She was fifty-years-old, overweight, and had been a lifelong dieter. She had tried every fad diet imaginable. She would lose weight from time to time but the second she stopped the "diet," the weight would come back on with gusto!

Sandy's labs when we started were diagnostic for metabolic syndrome. Her LDL was elevated, her HDL was low (37), her triglycerides were 151 (should be less than 100), her CRP (c-reactive protein a marker of inflammation) was >10 (should be <1), her fasting glucose was 110 (should be <90), fasting insulin was 23 (should be between 2-5), and her A1C, a three-month marker of glucose levels, was 8.8 (should be <5). She was the very image of metabolic dysfunction.

[9] Alam, I., Gul, R., Chong, J., Tan, C. T. Y., Chin, H. X., Wong, G., Doggui, R., & Larbi, A. (2019). Recurrent circadian fasting (RCF) improves blood pressure, biomarkers of cardiometabolic risk and regulates inflammation in men. Journal of Translational Medicine, 17(1). https://doi.org/10.1186/s12967-019-2007-z

Sandy's struggles with food were very real. It stopped being about hunger for her long ago. Food was a way to soothe her soul, and recently her soul needed a lot of soothing. Her marriage was failing. It was most likely the thing that tipped her over the edge and sealed her fate in terms of her breast cancer diagnosis.

For the first year following her diagnosis, Sandy dipped her toe into making some changes. She started by taking longer breaks between food from one day to the next. She made some better choices. She lost a little bit of weight, but she was far from her goal weight. Her marriage got worse. The holidays came and she went back to her self-soothing ways.

I heard from her six months later when she started to have back pain. Because the pain lasted for more than two weeks, and couldn't be otherwise explained, I asked her to get a study. Sadly, the study showed that Sandy's cancer had spread to her bones.

Sandy's new diagnosis terrified her—so much so that she was committed to finally taking control of her health once and for all. Sandy decided that while she was gathering all the information for how she would treat her recurrence, she would do a water fast.

She started with one day. That turned to two, then three. Before she knew it, she had fasted a week. Then two. A month went by where she consumed only water.

Here is what happened:
- She lost 20 lbs.
- Her fasting glucose went from 110 to 70.
- Her A1C and fasting insulin normalized.
- Her LDL dropped by 20 points.
- Her Triglycerides dropped to 90.
- The metabolic dysfunction corrected itself.

It's a miracle. Or is it?

You see the truth is, we are designed for fasting. It's when we are not living in accordance with our biology, when we are not living in accordance with nature and circadian rhythm, that our health suffers.

I know that Sandy's case is extreme. I am in no way implying you go a month without food. I just wanted to share with you the power that fasting has.

Fasting doesn't have to mean no food at all. In fact, the data on time restricted eating, intermittent fasting, and the fasting mimicking diet made famous by Dr. Valter Longo, is equally as impressive. There are ways of eating that can mimic a water fast allowing the consumption of food, during controlled time intervals, that allows people to get all the benefits of fasting without the total sacrifice.

We are modern beings living on a very old gene code. Our very existence is tied to circadian rhythm, the rhythm of the sun. We are meant to be active during the day and to rest safely at night. We are not meant to eat after dark. Our metabolism gets slower as the day goes on and really slows after dark. Therefore, to maintain a healthy metabolism, we need to focus on two things in terms of timing of eating. First, food should be consumed when the sun is out. Second, everyone benefits from a longer fast (three to seven days) several times a year to reset the system and allow for prolonged periods of healing. The way we prepare for those longer fasts is by extending our eating window from one day to the next so that we don't need to rely on a constant flow of calories. While this requires some training, it is by no means impossible. Once people get past a few days of time restricted eating and making better food choices, they find that they are not really hungry.

What Happens When We Fast?

Digestion actually takes a lot of work. When the body doesn't have to digest, it can get to the work of repairing itself. When we fast, and the body does not have its usual access to glucose, not only does it force the body to use fat cells for energy, but it also allows our cellular repair systems to get going! It is in the fasted state that our cellular repair mechanisms start to work efficiently. That means that if you are not fasting, your healing and repair mechanisms are not working as well as they should. This is a risk factor for disease. Overeating and eating too frequently prevent the body from repair and healing. It prevents the process called autophagy—the mechanism by which we repair and get rid of damaged or abnormal cells. Because of this, some degree of fasting is good for everyone, but there are people who should be particularly vigilant about fasting. There is considerable evidence to support fasting during chemotherapy treatment. In a study published in Therapeutic Advances in Medical Oncology, the fasting mimicking diet when used along with chemotherapy led to improved clinical response to neoadjuvant (up front) chemotherapy compared to a regular diet in HER2-negative early breast cancer patients receiving chemotherapy.[10]

When You Eat Matters

Why does eating frequently cause problems? Because eating is an inflammatory process. Did you know that 70% of our immune system is housed in the gut? It is charged with determining whether what comes into the gastrointestinal system is food or foe. This means that every single time you eat or drink, your immune system is obligated to investigate to see if this is something that is healthy and should be let into the system or is it something that is considered foreign or harmful, in which case the immune system responds with an immune response. What is that response? Inflammation!

Each time we eat, we are asking our immune system for a check in. Our immune system decides whether our food is friend or foe, which creates some degree of reaction to that food. Reaction = Inflammation. So, if we are eating one time a day, then that's happening once a day and how much inflammation is generated will largely depend on what you eat. If you're eating a very anti-inflammatory meal, then you're generating very little inflammation. Conversely, if you're eating every two or three hours (as many health professionals suggest) you're essentially in a constant inflammatory state. Grazers, or people eating tastes of food, here and there, all day long, are generating a near constant flow of inflammation. When you're grazing, your immune system never gets a

[10] Kikomeko, Joachim, Tim Schutte, M.J.M. Van Velzen, Rianne Seefat, and Hanneke W. M. Van Laarhoven. 2023. "Short-term Fasting and Fasting Mimicking Diets Combined With Chemotherapy: A Narrative Review." Therapeutic Advances in Medical Oncology (Print) 15 (January): 175883592311614. https://doi.org/10.1177/17588359231161418.

chance to rest. That inflammation is just building. As a result, you are more inflamed and vulnerable to the diseases associated with chronic inflammation, like breast cancer. Here's the rub. We all make cancer cells. Young, old, and everyone in between. An intact immune system should recognize those cells in their infancy and destroy them. However, if your immune system is so exhausted by having to examine a near constant flow of food and drink into the body, it is not going to be able to adequately defend against cancer development. Fasting, or periods of abstinence from food and calories, is the cornerstone of immune and metabolic health.

Food Is Inflammation

We know that each time we eat, it incites an inflammatory reaction. However, depending on what you eat, you may create more inflammation. There are many things that make food inflammatory. We just learned that frequent meals, or grazing, is one of the biggest sources of dietary inflammation. Processed foods are another. Since processed foods aren't real foods, the immune system doesn't recognize them as food and thus mounts an immune response. But even people who eat clean diets can have an immune response from food. Some of it is from food frequency, like we discussed. Some of it is due to the chemicals associated with our food. Some of it is from not chewing your food properly and it arrives at the small intestine in too large a mass to be recognized as its components. Some of it is a lack of acid or enzymes so the food fails to break down.

The Problem With Gluten

People with celiac disease have an immune reaction when they encounter wheat, or any of the gluten containing grains. I've even seen a connection between women with breast cancer who are later diagnosed with Celiac disease (and vice versa). But Celiac disease is only a small part of the gluten story. Non-Celiac gluten sensitivity is a huge source of inflammation. We know that chronic inflammation is the recipe for breast cancer. Gluten sensitivity is one of the most common causes of inflammation in our country. You see, we were not meant to consume grains. Grains are the seeds of grass. In order to digest grass, you need to have the gastrointestinal tract of a ruminator. Ruminators have long redundant gastrointestinal tracts, which are quite effective at extracting the nutrient from grains—they basically have two stomachs! Compared to ruminators, we have very short gastrointestinal tracts. For this reason, everyone struggles to some extent with digesting grains. Beyond that, though humans have been eating wheat for thousands of years, the wheat that we have in the United States is not the wheat of biblical times. The wheat in the United States is dwarf wheat, a genetically modified plant designed for far better seed yield. Einkorn wheat, the wheat of biblical times, has fourteen chromosomes. Modern wheat in the United States has forty-one chromosomes. Our genes have not caught up with our environment. Therefore, when eating wheat or any products made from wheat, we are challenging the immune system—gluten sensitive or not. (Please note this is not true for Europe. Europeans still use the wheat of biblical times that most of us have adapted to. In addition, the bread making process in Europe is a 24-48 hour process. In that time, most of the gluten has broken down. In the US, the average bread making process takes between two to four hours.) Compared to Celiac Disease, which is still relatively uncommon, Non-Celiac gluten sensitivity is a large issue for our society.

What happens when we ingest gluten? We induce a condition called intestinal permeability, or leaky gut. Our digestive tract is one long tube extending from the mouth to the anus. This tract is lined by cells that are attached to one another by tight junctions. The way we are supposed to absorb nutrients is by breaking down our food to the smallest of entities (amino acids, sugar, fatty acid). These then get absorbed through that single cell layer that lines our gut. When we ingest something inflammatory, the tight junctions open up and allow food to "leak" into the system. Technically, intact food or proteins are not supposed to cross that barrier. When they do, they come into direct contact with the immune system. This is how food sensitivity develops. This is the process of how we start to react to foods that we are not necessarily sensitive to.

It is for this reason that I often do not use food sensitivity testing until I heal the gut. People with leaky gut will respond to everything. Testing someone who actively has a leaky gut will be universally positive. It does nothing but create unnecessary anxiety and food avoidance.

Gluten is not the only trigger of intestinal permeability. We know that inflammatory states, chemotherapy, radiation, dairy, sugar, alcohol, caffeine, processed foods, food allergies, infections, dysbiosis (an unhealthy imbalance of the organisms housed in your gut), medications, long distance running, overexercise, and trauma also lead to intestinal permeability. Common medications associated with leaky gut are the NSAIDs (non-steroidal anti-inflammatory drugs like aspirin and ibuprofen), birth control pills, antibiotics, immunosuppressants, steroids, antacids, and acid blockers.

Wheat and grain sensitivity are certainly a problem. However, even if you are not sensitive to the grains themselves, consuming grains can still be quite inflammatory. Grains are notoriously laden with chemicals. Pesticides, herbicides, fungicides, and a well-known cancer-causing chemical called glyphosate are all coating your grain. These chemicals are deleterious to the microbiome, the ecosystem of organisms that exists in and on us. Our microbiome is intimately associated with our immune system. Our health is dependent on the health of our microbiome. Therefore, we need to be mindful of avoiding things that have a negative impact on it. Conventionally grown grains are amongst those foods that we all need to avoid.

The Problem with Dairy

The gluten story is only one example of how certain foods are inflammatory. Dairy is another. Because dairy is made by cows that consume grass (normally), the proteins in dairy resemble those in wheat. Therefore, there is a lot of crossover sensitivity between grains and dairy. This is one of the reasons that people who are gluten sensitive, or have celiac, should avoid dairy.

Even if you are not sensitive, another reason to avoid dairy stems around how the dairy cows are raised in the United States. Only a minority of dairy cows are pasture raised and exist on their native diet of grass. The vast majority of the cows in the US are raised commercially. Many are fed a diet of corn and soy, and as a result are highly inflamed themselves. They are given antibiotics to manage infections and antacids to stop them from regurgitating since their diet is artificial and they suffer horrible reflux. When we drink the milk of these cows, or eat their dairy products, not only are we reacting to their proteins that resemble grass, we are consuming their inflammatory byproducts. This is not a recipe for health.

Lastly, we must remember the purpose of cow's milk. Cow's milk is to make baby cows into big fat cows. It is loaded with growth hormones. Growth hormones are just about the last thing that someone with breast cancer needs more of, especially when it's coming from an inflamed cow.

Gluten and dairy sensitivity may very well be the reason why we see food allergies and sensitivities. Unfortunately, this creates a near constant feedback loop. As the food we eat causes intestinal permeability, our immune system gets triggered. It then releases histamine, which in turn causes more intestinal permeability. This can be a very frustrating position to be in.

The Problem with Processed Foods

And…we haven't even started to talk about processed foods. Again, we are modern beings living on a very old gene code. Our gut only recognizes real food, meaning that food had to have existed for thousands and thousands of years. When your body encounters an Oreo, a chocolate chip cookie, a slice of birthday cake, or even the protein powder that you use to make your smoothie, your immune system does not recognize that as food. So what happens? You get an inflammatory reaction. The more frequently you do that, the more inflamed you are. And so the cycle continues.

The Problem with Seed Oils

Another huge dietary source of inflammation is oils. We need a variety of fats to function optimally. However, the standard American diet is very heavily weighted toward inflammatory fats. Processed foods are laden with Omega 6's from highly processed oils. These include but are not limited to soybean, peanut, vegetable, safflower, canola, sunflower, corn, cottonseed, grape seed, rapeseed, and rice bran oil. These oils are manufactured utilizing high heat processes that oxidize the fats and cause them to be rancid. They must then undergo processes to eliminate the byproducts of that: bleaching to remove color pigments, and deodorization. Therefore, when we ingest these toxic oils, they create a toxicity in us.

By eliminating the major inflammatory foods, namely inflammatory oils and highly processed foods like bread, cereals, crackers, sugar, syrup, juice, corn syrup, artificial sweeteners, grains, dairy, commercially raised beef, pork, and poultry, farm-raised fish and shellfish, and instead replacing them with whole plant foods, you will materially change your health. What you take out is nearly as important as what you put in.

Secondary Foods

Food is not only calories and nutrients. Food is also information. The foods we eat not only inform our health, they inform the health of our microbiome, that ecosystem that lives in and on us. You cannot expect your body to put out intelligent work when you are feeding it a diet devoid of quality information.

From a genetic standpoint, we are only 10% human. That means that 90% of our genetic information comes from our microbiome. The majority of our microbiome resides in our gut. When we feed our microbiome with good information, or good food, it relays good information to our body. However, the converse is also true. Poor information undoubtedly leads to poor performance. My mommy always told me you are what you eat and what you eat matters. The fact that she fed me Doritos and Fig Newtons on a daily basis is a story for another time.

Seventy percent of our microbiome lives in our digestive tract, as does 70% of our immune system. Our microbiome is in constant communication and contact with our immune system, and is responsible for our cravings, the things that we want to eat. Cravings are signals from your microbiome. They are asking you for what they want or need. So if you have a microbiome made up of sugar eaters, because you fed them a diet of sugar, then that's what you will crave. A microbiome of sugar eaters will not convey healthy information to your immune system and your health will suffer.

Conversely, if you have broccoli eaters, kale, eaters, and colorful vegetable eaters, that's what you're going to crave. They are full of good information which will be relayed to your immune system.

Your Microbiome Can Change

For many years, more than I wish to admit, I was addicted to birthday cake. I thought it was a food group. I would be the mom that would order the biggest cake you could acceptably order for your kid's birthday, make sure that all the kids got a piece of it, and then eat the rest of it myself. I loved birthday cake. I remember the sense of accomplishment that I felt after I had changed my entire diet and the way I ate. I went from the person that could absolutely not resist a piece of cake to the person I am now that doesn't even take a bite. These days, if you had put a bowl of steaming kale with onions and garlic and mushrooms in front of me, I would recommend you watch your fingers because I would gobble it up. I share this story so that you can appreciate the fact that your microbiome, and what it eats, can change. When you stop eating sugar, and all the food-like substances that don't nourish you, the microbes that eat sugar or junk food die off, and they're replaced with the microbes that eat whatever you replace the sugar and junk food with! The good news about that is that your microbiome can always be changed by what you eat, and sometimes pretty rapidly. That's why our genes are only a small part of what happens to our health. The true story lies in the microbiome and the genes that they have, because, basically, we are borrowing our health—good, bad or indifferent, from our microbiome.

So What Do I Eat?

Now, I'm sure you're wondering what you should actually eat! This is probably the biggest part of the breast cancer journey for most people. I want to be clear that it's super important, but it's not everything. I try to, as much as I can, discourage orthorexia (an obsession with diets). Diet isn't religion. I don't want you so strict about your food that you are not enjoying life. Your diet shouldn't be a source of stress and distress. This is what we're trying to get rid of. I want you to adopt as much as you can, but I also want to be clear that it needs to make sense and feel good for you.

In her book, Radical Remission, Kelly Turner identifies nine key factors she witnessed in people who underwent a "spontaneous remission." As you likely know by now, their remission wasn't truly spontaneous because they were taking actions to eliminate toxins and improve their health. The main thing all of these people did was change their diet.

Before we go any further, let me emphasize that your diet shouldn't be a source of stress. I want you to enjoy life, while also understanding and cultivating eating habits that support you on your journey to heal. Adopt what you can, but do what makes sense and feels good for you. In the words of Hippocrates, "Let food be thy medicine and medicine be thy food."

The Anti-Breast Cancer Diet

I again want to reiterate there's no one diet that's right for everyone with breast cancer. If there were, there would be no role for our 800-billion-dollar diet industry. People talk about all kinds of different diets: an alkaline diet, the Paleo diet, the Keto diet, but the bottom line is that when we're talking about an anti-cancer diet, we are talking about a whole food plant rich diet. That is because the way we eat, the things that we eat, have a profound effect on what happens to us on a cellular level.

We discussed before that we are all reproducing cells, all the time. Inevitably, we are going to make mistakes in that process. Or our cells will get exposed to something that damages them. We need cellular repair mechanisms to guard against the things in our environment that damage our cells. That is where your diet comes in. You want to consume a diet that supports these repair mechanisms AND protects you from your environment.

What you eat can turn on and off the genes that influence the progression and regression of cancer. Different foods have their own unique anti-cancer effect on our body. When you eat things like arugula, watercress and kale, the phytonutrients in them suppress cancer cell growth. Spinach, asparagus, beets, and lentils are all rich in B vitamins. The B vitamins are essential to the synthesis and repair of DNA. Vitamin C acts as a powerful antioxidant. You will find Vitamin C in red peppers, strawberries, citrus fruits, Brussels sprouts, kale, broccoli, and papaya.

Michael Pollan summarized all dietary theory into this one statement: "Eat real food. Not too much, mostly plants."

If there is one theory that applies to everyone, this is what it is. Now, I have come up with what I believe is the ideal plan for people who are trying to prevent a breast cancer diagnosis, who are living with breast cancer, or are preventing the return or the recurrence of breast cancer.

Here is the anti-breast cancer diet: It is a whole food, plant based, grain free, low glycemic diet.

In order to get started, let's talk about the components of the diet and the way you will create your meal plan. There are five food groups that are so nutrient dense, so important, that they should be included in your diet every day. They are:

- Leafy greens
- Cruciferous vegetables
- Onions
- Mushrooms
- Garlic

These are the foods that you are going to make sure you consume on a daily basis.

Leafy greens include kale, collards, spinach, chard, escarole, etc. They are loaded with antioxidants that can neutralize free radicals from things like radiation, and therefore prevent cancer. In a 2012 study published in the Journal of the National Cancer Institute, researchers found that women who ate dark, leafy greens had a far lower breast cancer risk than the women who didn't.

Cruciferous vegetables include broccoli, broccoli sprouts, cauliflower, Brussels sprouts, cabbage, and Bok Choy. My kids call these the stinky vegetables, as they are high in sulfur content. They contain a substance called sulforaphane, which helps the body with detoxification.

Then there's the onion family. That includes onions, shallots, anise, fennel, scallions, chives and leeks. These vegetables have high levels of quercetin, fisetin, and Vitamin C. They serve to inhibit proliferation or cell growth, reduce migration and invasiveness, and induce apoptosis in human breast cancer cells. Consuming onions in your daily diet can also make cancer cells less resistant to therapies.

Garlic is in a class of its own and should be consumed daily. It has been demonstrated to prevent breast cancer growth and progression at all its stages.

Lastly is the mushroom family. Though all mushrooms have medicinal value, the medicinal mushrooms are practically magical. Mushrooms are the detoxifiers of the forest and everything they do in nature, they do in you. They take rotting organic matter and turn it into the beautiful fruiting body that we consume. They aid in digestion, respiratory health, blood sugar balance, lower blood pressure and help to maintain metabolic health. They help with sleep, are anti-inflammatory, and protect against depression and anxiety. They are antiviral, antibacterial and antifungal. They are also known for their anti-cancer properties. Many mushrooms are natural aromatase inhibitors (as are cabbage, kale, Brussels sprouts, onions and garlic, citrus fruits, apples, and parsley due to their quercetin content). All of these foods are extremely helpful in terms of hormone balance. The medicinal mushrooms include lion's mane, shiitake, maitake, chaga, cordyceps, reishi and turkey tail. There are books and books written about the medicinal properties of mushrooms and I recommend including them in your diet or supplement routine every day!

How to Prepare Food on the Anti-Breast Cancer Diet

I have some preparation tips in order to get the most out of these foods. It is important to chop onions and garlic ten minutes before their use or consumption to activate their enzymes. Roasting whole garlic cloves, while delicious, robs you of its benefits. Kale needs massaging to start to break it down and broccoli needs chopping forty minutes before eating or cooking. Lastly, mushrooms should never be consumed raw. Their medicinal value is only available when they are heated.

The key to microbiome and gut health is diversity. So, in addition to these five groups, you need to make sure that you are eating a rainbow of plant foods over the course of the week. You do not need to eat each color every day, but you should be covering the colors weekly.

I advocate for a variety of raw and cooked foods, as both have their values. If you are unaccustomed to eating a lot of vegetables, there is no time like the present to get going. Start slow and build up. Eventually, you will be like me and drool at the thought of them. If you need to add digestive enzymes until your body is accustomed to eating these foods, I suggest you do that.

The biggest concern people have when they adopt a plant-based diet is that they aren't getting enough protein, or they're worried about controlling their macros. Everything has protein in it. Being aware of plant-based foods that contain more protein will help you to reach your goals. Things like tofu, pumfu, beans and legumes will help you to meet your protein needs while satisfying you and providing fiber for detoxification. Remember, food is medicine. Food is information. When we give the body what it needs, the body functions optimally.

I believe that people should listen to the signals of their body and eat when they're hungry. For some people, that is going to be once a day. Others, that is twice or three times. Each time you eat, if you plan your plate accordingly, you will meet your protein, fat, and fiber needs. Those are the important ones to ensure long term health. Tune into how you feel. Are you getting enough, and does what you're eating make you feel good? These are really important questions that need answers. Also, diets change. Eating patterns change. What and when you eat changes seasonally and with age. As we get older, we need more protein to maintain muscle mass but not so much that we are encouraging tumor growth. This is about balance and dialing in to how you feel. Remember what you learned about fasting though and plan accordingly. If you eat properly at your meals, there should be no need for snacking or grazing. Meals should ideally be consumed during daylight hours and your smallest meal should be at the end of the day.

When you eat, you should divide your plate into three to four parts. For those actively cancering, three quarters of your plate should be filled with non-starchy vegetables. The remaining quarter should be protein. You should never be consuming more than five to six ounces of protein in one meal. Our bodies are only capable of digesting so much protein at a time. Excess protein consumption will only lead to increased fat storage and glucose production. This has the exact opposite effect to what you are looking for.

Other Important Frequent Foods

I would be totally remiss if I wrote a book about breast cancer and didn't address the issue around soy. Soy, and other phyto - or plant estrogens get a terrible rap. This is because of the widespread misconception that estrogen causes breast cancer. In the words of the brilliant Dr. William Li, "It's time to overturn that urban legend." In his book, Eat To Beat Disease, he states:

Phytoestrogens in soy do not increase the incidence of breast cancer in human studies. Soy phytoestrogens actually act as antiestrogens in humans and can activate tumor suppressor genes.

Additionally, the genistein in soy has antiangiogenic, cancer-starving effects. I consider soy to be a superfood and recommend its consumption regularly. I am also careful about the kinds of soy that I recommend. Soy should be unprocessed (edamame) or minimally processed (soy milk, tofu, miso, tempeh, natto), organic, and non-GMO. I am not a fan of highly processed soy products. Soy protein isolate doesn't benefit anyone.

I put flax in a similar category to soy. Flaxseed is the richest dietary source of lignans, a type of phytoestrogen. Researchers have shown that flaxseed sprouts can increase apoptosis (programmed cell death). Some cell and animal studies have shown that two specific phytoestrogens found in lignans, named enterolactone and enterodiol, may help suppress breast tumor growth. Animal studies have shown that both flaxseed oil and lignans can reduce breast tumor growth and spread, even for ER-cancer cells.[11] This result suggests that flaxseeds may have anti-cancer benefits that are unrelated to any type of effect on estrogen or estrogen metabolism. There are studies that show that ground flaxseed can reduce tumor growth in both breast and prostate cancer. Flax has favorable effects on insulin and insulin like growth factors which can improve metabolic health and make a hostile environment for cancer. I recommend two tablespoons of ground flax every day. I love to sprinkle mine on my soup, my salad, or mix it in with my chia pudding.

Coffee contains a large amount of polyphenols. As such, it has been found to be both protective against the development of breast cancer and associated with decreased recurrence and all cause mortality after breast cancer.[12] So if you're a coffee drinker, drink up! Just make sure that it's organic and mold-free. My favorite coffee is infused with medicinal mushrooms. I call it my functional medicine in a cup! You can find my coffee and other recommendations in the resource guide at the end of this book.

Green tea is another breast cancer obstacle. The bioactives in green tea include catechins like ECGC, flavonols, phenolic acids, and methylxanthines. These chemicals ignite the activity of our tumor suppressor genes enhancing the body's ability to avoid or reverse cancer.

[11] Flaxseed. Natural Medicines Comprehensive Database. Accessed March 24, 2013

[12] Nehlig, Astrid, Nathalie Reix, Pauline Arbogast, and Carole Mathelin. 2021. "Coffee Consumption and Breast Cancer Risk: A Narrative Review in the General Population and in Different Subtypes of Breast Cancer." European Journal of Nutrition 60 (3): 1197–1235. https://doi.org/10.1007/s00394-020-02465-0.

In addition to its epigenetic or gene-activating properties, green tea is known for its association with lowering blood pressure, blood sugar and cholesterol. Perhaps that is one of the mechanisms with which green tea helps with breast cancer as it serves to improve metabolic health. To get the most out of your green tea, I recommend drinking matcha which is made from the ground unfermented leaves of the plant Camellia Sinensis. If you don't have sensitivity to caffeine, as green tea does have some, I recommend four cups a day. Decaffeinated green tea, for those that are sensitive, can be just as beneficial.

Selenium, found in things like brazil nuts, is a nutrient that is tied to the health of a number of our body systems. In a recent study of breast cancer patients in Poland, selenium levels were found to directly correlate with long term survival. Those with the highest selenium levels had a 20% increase in survival compared to those with the lowest levels.[13] To get your daily dose of selenium, I recommend eating two Brazil nuts every day. Other good sources of selenium include lentils, mushrooms and sunflower seeds.

This is your foundation. This is the habit to be built, and it won't be automatic. It's something that's going to need to be practiced, just like any other habit. For the first few weeks that you're doing this, you're probably going to need a checklist with you. I have included your weekly checklist in the Resources section at the end of this book. Over time, it will become more and more innate.

Five Goals to a Healthier, Happier You

Here are your goals to get on the road to a healthier, happier you:

> 1. **Aim to consume six to nine cups of non-starchy vegetables a day.** When I say non-starchy, I mean no potatoes, root vegetables, etc. Instead, you should be eating water-based vegetables. People always say to me, "That is a tremendous amount of vegetables!" And I say, "Yes that's

[13] Szwiec, Marek, Wojciech Marciniak, Róża Derkacz, Tomasz Huzarski, Jacek Gronwald, Cezary Cybulski, Tadeusz Dębniak, et al. 2021. "Serum Selenium Level Predicts 10-Year Survival After Breast Cancer." Nutrients 13 (3): 953. https://doi.org/10.3390/nu13030953.

true." The intention is that if you're so focused on getting these vegetables, the likelihood that you're going to take in things that don't serve you, that don't promote your health, is very low. Not only do they fill you, they also crowd out those other things that are not good for you.

2. **Include those five groups of vegetables daily.** the leafy greens, the cruciferous, the onions, the garlic, and the mushrooms.

3. **Include ground flax, green tea, and selenium every day.**

4. **Fill your plate with mostly vegetables and a five-ounce portion of protein.** Be sure to include a source of healthy fat on your vegetables. Things like olive oil, avocado, nuts and seeds are great additions and sources of healthy fat. Fat and protein are what keep us satiated and satisfied.

5. **Get most of your "colors" from vegetables.** The blacks and the blues are hard to do, so it's okay to include dark berries if that is where you are going to get your anthocyanins. Just remember that the evolutionary purpose of fruit was to make us fat during the summer so that we could survive the scarcity during the winter. As we no longer have winter, and no longer have scarcity, we no longer have a need for year-long fructose. Your body knows what season it is, so in as much as you can, eat locally and seasonally. If you are consuming fruit, you should be consuming no more than one cup or one serving a day. Fruits and vegetables are defined by their color. Remember when you're choosing your vegetables that you want the strongest color possible. The pigment in the plant is protecting that plant from the forces of nature, and you want that same benefit in you. Whenever picking a plant, go for color.

Other Things to Remember

Fermented foods are rich in probiotics and very good for your microbiome. Try to include some of them on a weekly basis. Opt for low sugar options like fermented vegetables. Kombucha and kefir are delicious, but many of them are so high in sugar that it negates the benefit for you.

Eliminate sugar in all its forms as it is highly inflammatory and your body can make all the sugar it needs. This includes juice. While there might be nutrients in juice, I believe the fiber is most important and you lose all of that in the process of juicing. (Technically, the juice cleanse suggested at the beginning of this book is a fast and meant to be short-term. I do not believe in long-term juicing.)

Give up grains, even if you are not sensitive. Our bodies have no nutritional need for grains. If we never ate another grain again, we would suffer no nutritional deficiency. Everyone is healthier when they eliminate grains from their diet.

All animal protein is inflammatory. If you are going to eat animals, make sure they are raised in the most natural way possible. Think pasture raised, grass-fed meat and poultry, and wild, line-caught fish.

Get to know the EWG Clean 15 and Dirty Dozen so you know which foods you need to purchase organic and which ones can safely be consumed even if they were grown commercially. Know that you are not going to be perfect and pretty good is often great!

Foods That Inhibit Aromatase Activity

The following foods contain compounds that have been shown to inhibit aromatase activity, thereby suppressing excess estrogen biosynthesis. Before you do too much to decrease your endogenous (self) production of estrogen, I would make sure to eliminate as many environmental estrogens, or xenoestrogens, as you can. A full list of xenoestrogens can be found in the toxin section of this book. They include things like plastics, plasticizers, non-stick coatings, fragrance, perfumes, antibiotics, and other such substances.

- Artichokes
- Arugula
- Blueberries & bilberries
- Broccoli & broccoli sprouts
- Brussels sprouts
- Cabbage
- Cauliflower
- Celery
- Cherries, sour or tart
- Chives
- Cilantro
- Collard greens
- Cox -2 inhibitors (EPA,curcumin)
- Chrysin
- Cranberries & lingonberries
- Currants, black
- Dietary Fiber
- Grapes, red
- Grape seed extract
- Green onions
- Green tea
- Horseradish & wasabi
- Hot peppers
- Iodine
- Isoflavones from soy
- Kale
- Lemons & limes
- Lignans from flax seed
- Mexican oregano
- Mushrooms, white button & related
- Mustard
- Mustard greens
- Oranges & tangerines
- Parsley
- Pomegranates
- Progesterone
- Radishes
- Resveratrol
- Rice (black, red| or purple)
- Saffron
- Turnip greens
- Turnips
- Walnuts & walnut oil
- Watercress
- White button mushrooms

The Fasting Mimicking Diet

For anyone deciding to undergo chemotherapy, perhaps the most important tool you need is the Fasting Mimicking Diet. This way of eating convinces your body that you are fasting while still being able to enjoy some food. This is of great benefit in terms of patient compliance when compared to a three-day water fast. Fasting while getting chemotherapy is very important as it allows the body to protect the normal cells while making the cancer cells even more vulnerable. The research on this coming from Dr. Valter Longo and others is very promising. The following is a guide to the Fasting Mimicking Diet.

GOALS: Low calorie, low glycemic, high fat eating plan to be consumed 1-2 days prior to and the day of chemotherapy. Resume your anticancer diet the day after chemotherapy.

Eat two meals a day. Each meal consists of:
- One-half an avocado or a handful of mixed nuts (Brazil/almonds/pistachios/walnuts)
- One green smoothie (cucumber, celery, dandelion greens, spinach, kale, lemon, ginger in a blender) or one scoop of Bulletproof[14] or Indigo greens mixed with water or 1.5 cups of homemade, grain-free, potato-free vegetable soup

Daily Snacks:
- 10 Olives
- 5 seed crackers (Flackers or Ella's Flats)

Be sure to drink 60 oz. of filtered water and four cups of green, ginger, cilantro or parsley tea daily. Hydration during this time is of the utmost importance.

Note: Before starting any fasting routine, please discuss this with your physician. People who already have muscle wasting will need to add bone broth or a source of protein to this regimen.

How You Eat Matters

I'll finish this chapter by talking about how we eat, because with all nourishment, you need to be in a place to receive it. Just like people can show you great kindness and say wonderful things to you, if you're not in a place to receive it, it has no effect. It's the same exact thing with food. If you're not in a place to receive those nutrients, if you're running around eating on the go, if you are focused on something else and you're not in a calm parasympathetic state, then you're not going to be able to

---

[14] https://tinyurl.com/RHMDbulletproofgreens

digest your food. If you're not in a parasympathetic rest and digest state, you're not going to be able to extract and absorb the nutrient the way that you're supposed to. How we eat is as important as what we eat and when we eat. So, I need you to really think about how you are eating your meals. Are you sitting down? Are you focused on your food? Are you grateful for that meal and for the food that you're about to receive? Are you in a non-distracted place without a screen of some kind? How we eat, the state in which we eat, the intentions we set before we eat, all play a major role in how we receive our food. It is as important as when and what we eat.

When you put this all together, you have the recipe for gut health. That alone will get you more than halfway toward your health goals.

Everything we eat is either lifting us up or pulling us down. The food we eat and the water that we drink is either making us healthy or sick. Knowing what not to eat can sometimes be every bit as important as knowing what to eat. It's imperative to know the things that trigger inflammation and trigger stress chemistry and knowing what and how to eat to calm or avoid inflammation. As I have stated before, I do not think that there is one diet, one set of foods, that is the key to reversing cancer. But there are guidelines to follow that will materially improve your health, significantly diminish inflammation, and consciously create the chemistry of joy.

For anyone who is cancering, here is probably the most important concept for you to understand. Health happens at home. There is no kitchen outside of your home that is going to care about the quality of your food as much as you do. I am not saying that you'll never have another meal out. However, if health is truly your goal then the majority of the food that you consume will most likely need to be prepared in your home. This is not to say that you can't enjoy an occasional meal out. However, most restaurants prepare their food with ingredients that are the least expensive. But cheap food is very costly—to you and your health. In the resource section in the back, you will find a guide to the foods that you should try to eat every day, try to eat every week, and the foods to avoid. It would behoove you to get that list now, and go through your kitchen getting rid of as many of the no items as you can. Replace them with the staples on the YES list and set yourself up for success.

What Nourishes Us?

We all know that what everyone needs at the end of the day is nourishment. What we don't really think about is where that nourishment comes from. In this book, I discuss the foods that will nourish you throughout your cancer journey and beyond. But I would be remiss if I didn't really define nourishment for you.

At the very start of my healing journey, I mentioned that I attended IIN, the Institute for Integrative Nutrition. Joshua Rosenthal founded this institution on this monumental theory: Nourishment consists of two separate categories: primary food and secondary food. Most people believe that what they put in their mouths is primary food. However, this is flawed thinking. The primary things that nourish us do not have caloric content at all.

We can live a very long time without food. That has been proven time and time again in history. Gandhi fasted for twenty-one days in protest of violence and the inequities of his society. The body is capable of amazing things. But here are the things that we can't survive without. These things are actually our *primary* food.

- Regular physical movement
- Meaningful positive relationships
- Fulfilling work
- Some form of spiritual connection (whatever that is for you)
- Joy
- Non-dietary forms of self-care
- Playfulness, creativity, and fun
- Purpose
- Sunshine
- Touch
- Love

The primary things that nourish us are what really fill our cups. This is our motivation for living and it's these very things that are described in the books called Radical Remission and Radical Hope by Kelly Turner. These are the very things that make you feel alive that actually keep you alive. If you are to survive and thrive following this dreadful diagnosis, it is a focus on these things that will propel you towards health.

What if we actually prioritized the things that nourished us? What if we actually prioritized primary food? What if we made sure to incorporate all those primary foods, things like forest bathing, taking walks in nature, and being connected on a daily basis to the ground and the earth? What if we prioritize our relationships, and make sure that our lives are filled with hugs and physical touch? What if we made sure that we had exposure to sunlight every day? Do you think if we did that we would still be so hungry? I am reminded so often of people using food to fill a void. They use food because they are not getting primary nourishment. They are not getting those primary foods.

This was definitely the case for Sandy. Sandy used secondary food to attempt to nourish herself. Unfortunately, all that led to was weight gain, hormone imbalance, metabolic decline, and breast cancer.

I want you to take a moment and think about what's nourishing you. Contemplate this concept of primary and secondary food knowing that secondary food is what you put in your mouth, and primary food is what truly nourishes you. What do your primary foods look like? Take time to examine your relationships. What makes you joyful? What kind of movement makes you happy? How much fresh air are you enjoying every day? How often are you enjoying the warm sun on your skin? How often are you appreciating the beauty that surrounds us in nature, the love that you have for your spouse or your child? It's the random acts of kindness done for us and by us for others that fuel our health. There are many great people who exemplified just this. The father of the Jewish people, Abraham, and his wife Sarah generously and lovingly provided food and shelter to those in need. Martin Luther King lived a life in service for others. Despite the hate that surrounded him, his soul was filled with love. It was his service to others that nourished him until that moment when he took his last breath. You don't need to be a historical giant to reap these benefits. By simply practicing gratitude for the simple things in life, you nourish your soul. We are nourished by countless things. By our connections to one another, our connections to family, to friends, and to our larger community, to God, and to the Universe. We are nourished by nature, our connection with nature, and being in sync with nature. There are endless sources of primary foods. We just need to prioritize them.

From here on in, I encourage you to make primary foods every bit as much a priority as secondary foods.

Action Items:
- Start a fasting practice.
- Eat an anti-inflammatory diet.
- Eat in a way that you can be nourished.
- Get your primary foods every day.

CHAPTER SEVEN - THE JOYS OF MOVEMENT

Exercise is the best medicine and is essential to both reversal and long-term remission from cancer. In her book, Radical Hope, Kelly Turner found exercise to be one of the key factors that led to a "radical remission." She interviewed thousands of "terminal" cancer patients (we're all terminal by the way) who were told that their breast cancer was an incurable disease. Those that got their disease to go into remission all have this in common: They added movement or exercise back into their lives as soon as they were strong enough to do so. Even for those that at the time of their treatment were too weak to begin a movement program, if they began to move once they were strong enough, they saw progress. They healed. By engaging in some type of movement, this effort shifted the course of their healing process. Any physical activity is better than none. A sedentary lifestyle is in part responsible for the decline of human health. Many Americans have a lifestyle of sitting, lying around, or just not moving the body. This type of lifestyle leads to cellular degeneration, muscle loss, loss of metabolic health, and the increased risk of cardiovascular disease and cancer. The body was made to move. If we do not engage in some type of physical activity it will begin to break down. The deal with the body is this: If you don't move it, you lose it!

All of that is to say, the functional medicine approach to cancer treatment involves exercising. Here's Why:

First of all, cancer hates oxygen. Cancer thrives in a hypoxic state. It gets its energy from anaerobic processes (anaerobic means without air). So, the more movement you do, the more movement you can do. While doing said movement, you are increasing your circulation and increasing your respiration and oxygenation. This results in the delivery of nutrients to the cells and delivery of the cells that help with cancer cell surveillance, destruction, and cellular health.

Exercise is so important that The American Society of Clinical Oncology (ASCO) released guidelines in 2022 to provide guidance on exercise, diet, and weight management during active cancer treatment in adults. Their decision was based on evidence from forty-two systematic reviews and an additional twenty-three randomized controlled trials. They stated:

Exercise during cancer treatment led to improvements in cardiorespiratory fitness, strength, fatigue, and other patient-reported outcomes. Preoperative exercise in patients with lung cancer led to a reduction in postoperative length of hospital stay and complications.[15]

Ultimately, their recommendations were that Oncology providers should recommend regular aerobic and resistance exercise during active treatment with curative intent.

Research on Exercise Prescription for Americans

Research from the Surgeon General (2008) recommends that all Americans over the age of six engage in 150 minutes of moderate exercise or seventy-five minutes of vigorous exercise per week. Further, the 2018 Physical Activity Guidelines for Americans concluded that everyone's health improves with physical activity and mandates that adults with chronic conditions and disabilities like cancer should avoid inactivity, at all costs.[16] They also said,

---

[15] Ligibel, Jennifer A., et al. 2022. "Exercise, Diet, and Weight Management During Cancer Treatment: ASCO Guideline." Journal of Clinical Oncology 40 (22): 2491–2507. https://doi.org/10.1200/jco.22.00687.
[16] Piercy, Katrina L., et. al.. 2018. "The Physical Activity Guidelines for Americans." JAMA 320 (19): 2020. https://doi.org/10.1001/jama.2018.14854.

A single bout of moderate-to-vigorous physical activity can improve that night's sleep, reduce anxiety symptoms, improve cognition, reduce blood pressure, and improve insulin sensitivity on the day that it is performed".[17] Over time, these benefits of exercise help to establish and maintain metabolic health which helps both reverse and prevent cancer. It's a win-win situation![18]

These are really powerful words, right? They are coming directly from our government and yet they are not included in most medical treatment plans. Exercise Medicine is not part of treatment paradigms. We hardly talk about it! Why? Probably because it can't be monetized. We have mastered the art of sending mixed messages and creating confusion among patients and medical professionals alike. We don't talk about exercise in the context of reversing cancer because it makes the doctors feel uncomfortable. Doctors like to be involved in the process, and exercise basically takes them out of it. In addition, this is never a part of physician training and so there is an inherent belief that it is either untrue or unimportant.

Additionally, obesity is a global epidemic and is the number one cause of preventable deaths in America. Obesity poses a direct and severe cancer risk. Obesity and inactivity often go hand in hand with one another. However, a contributing root cause of both cancer and obesity is inflammation. Inflammation in the body is decreased by exercise and movement.

Inflammation can become chronic if the cause of the inflammation persists or certain control mechanisms in charge of shutting down the process fail. When these inflammatory responses become chronic, cell mutation and proliferation can result, often creating an environment that is conducive to the development of cancer.[19]

---

[17] https://health.gov/sites/default/files/2019-09/PAG_Advisory_Committee_Report.pdf
[18] "The Physical Activity Guidelines"
[19] Singh N, Baby D, Rajguru JP, Patil PB, Thakkannavar SS, Pujari VB. Inflammation and cancer. Ann Afr Med. 2019 Jul-Sep;18(3):121-126. doi: 10.4103/aam.aam_56_18. PMID: 31417011; PMCID: PMC6704802.

There are many scientifically proven benefits of exercise. Here are a few:

- Exercise reduces the risk of dying prematurely.
- Exercise reduces inflammation.
- Exercise reduces the risk of dying from heart disease or cancer.
- Exercise reduces the risk of developing diabetes and high blood pressure.
- Exercise reduces blood pressure and lowers blood sugar, which is why it prevents diabetes and high blood pressure.
- Exercise reduces feelings of depression and anxiety.
- Exercise is equal or better at controlling depression than any drug on the market today.
- Exercise improves sleep, body image, and self esteem.
- Exercise, when performed correctly, does not have negative side effects, especially when compared to pharmaceutical drugs.

Exercise During Treatment

Exercise has many positive benefits for your health and healing journey. It can help you to maintain healthy weight because of all the other beneficial things it brings to your life. It also helps you to maintain healthy bones, muscles, joints, and ligaments. Exercise extends your lifespan. This goes way beyond just burning calories. Exercise is a game changer—it is medicine. It is universally effective and contributes to long term health benefits of all populations of people.

Research from the highly touted American College of Sports Medicine decisively concluded that exercise is not only safe and feasible during cancer treatment, but can improve physical functioning, reduce fatigue, and enhance quality of life during treatment. Cancer patients who exercise are stronger than those who don't. Studies at Dana Farber Cancer Institute have shown that exercise may help reduce the risk of recurrence in cancer patients. It has also been shown to help elevate mood, reduce anxiety, improve sleep, boost energy, and help reduce symptoms of treatment-related side effects, such as neuropathy.

A Brigham and Women's Hospital study shows that a brisk walking program nearly cut in half the risk of early death in breast cancer patients. In a similar study published in Brain, Behavior, and Immunity, those individuals who exercised had reduced levels of inflammatory markers in their blood, like C-Reactive Protein (CRP) and Tumor Necrosis Factor (TNF).[20] They were also able to maintain neurocognitive function, which correlates to decreased inflammation in the blood, leading to decreased inflammation in the brain. This is one way of preventing "chemo brain." If there are less inflammatory factors circulating around, there is less inflammation. Chemo brain is one of the biggest side effects that people report when they get chemotherapy. Cancer patients also experience a similar brain compromising phenomenon with anti-hormonal drugs, as estrogen is protective of brain function and the loss of estrogen is accompanied by a loss of cognitive function, difficulty with recall, mood disturbance, sleep disruption, and more. (We'll cover this in greater detail in Chapter 15.)

Exercise improves fatigue and pain levels. Many people have trouble getting started with an exercise routine and they make excuses for not exercising. One excuse is that they say they are too tired to exercise. However, it is the lack of exercise that makes them tired in the first place. The less you do the less you can do. That works conversely too!

Exercise and Metabolism

Cancer cells rewire their metabolism to promote growth, survival, proliferation, and long-term maintenance. This altered metabolism results in increased glucose uptake and fermentation of glucose to lactate. This is an anaerobic process known as the Warburg Effect. The Warburg Effect has been documented for over ninety years and extensively studied over the past twenty years with thousands of papers detailing this

---

[20] Khosravi, Nasim, Lee Stoner, Vahid Farajivafa, and Erik D. Hanson. 2019. "Exercise Training, Circulating Cytokine Levels and Immune Function in Cancer Survivors: A Meta-analysis." Brain, Behavior, and Immunity 81 (October): 92–104. https://doi.org/10.1016/j.bbi.2019.08.187.

process. Exercise lowers blood glucose therefore decreasing the amount of glucose that is available to cancer cells. In lowering glucose, we also lower insulin, reducing inflammation and lowering insulin resistance. Insulin is a hormone produced by the pancreas that is released in the bloodstream following a rise in blood sugar. We know that one of the roles of insulin is that it acts as a growth hormone. Growth hormone is the last thing that anyone with breast cancer needs. High levels of insulin set off a growth cascade. The more insulin we make, the less sensitive we are to that insulin, which means we need even more to have an effect. The more insulin we make, the more insulin-like growth factor (IGF-1) we make. The more IGF-1, the more growth there is. IGF-1 has been identified as both causing breast cancer and increasing the risk of recurrence.[21] This forward feeding loop of elevated blood sugar, high insulin, and IGF-1 leads to very poor metabolic health and breast cancer progression. Exercise lowers glucose and insulin levels. Weight training in particular can help to build muscle, increase your basal metabolic rate, increase your ratio of lean muscle to fat, lower blood sugar, lower insulin, and therefore help you to achieve metabolic health. Metabolic health is the key to reversing cancer!

Exercise and The Immune System

Exercise has the power to increase your immune cell count and productivity. Anyone who is taking prescription medications that lowers white blood cell count (which includes nearly all the drugs used to treat breast cancer) can improve their white cell count by exercising. White blood cells help the body heal and protect us against infections and diseases. Specifically, exercise helps with the formation of natural killer cells, the cells that directly attack cancer cells. As cancer is a failure of the immune system, most people already have a challenged immunity BEFORE they get breast cancer. Immune failure for many is one of the reasons why they got breast cancer. It's whatever made the immune

---

[21] "Insulin-like growth factor-1 (IGF-1), insulin growth factor-binding protein-3 (IGFBP-3) and breast cancer risk: observational and Mendelian randomization analyses with ~430,000 women", by Neil Murphy et al. Annals of Oncology.

system fail that allowed breast cancer to happen. The many drugs people with breast cancer are placed on further lower immunity, and only serve to complicate the problem. While you are figuring out your why, exercise can start to restore the health of your immune system.

Exercise and The Lymphatic System

Exercise increases lymphatic flow through the lymphatic system and works to keep your bodily fluids flowing properly. The lymph system is both your immune system and your detoxification system. The Lymphatic System has three main jobs. First, it clears excess fluids from the cells. Second, it absorbs fatty acids and helps to transport fats throughout the bloodstream. Third, it produces the lymphocytes, monocytes, and other antibody cells called plasma cells. To ensure the health of the immune system, you must have proper lymphatic flow. Movement and muscle use are the way that you do that. Rebounding, or jumping on a trampoline, is an especially great way to improve lymphatic circulation and your overall health while exercising. It's wonderful to layer things that have synergistic positive effects. We'll talk more about rebounding in Chapter 12.

Exercise and Digestion

Exercise improves gut barrier function. As we discussed earlier, this allows for nutrients to be absorbed without breaching the lining of the gut. The cells that line our gut are tightly adherent to one another. However, inflammation and certain foods can adversely affect gut barrier function. When the cells open and allow food to come across the barrier, it is then introduced to our immune system and sets off an inflammatory cascade. This causes inflammation due to the food coming into direct contact with the immune system of the gut. Exercise helps to tighten those junctions between the cells. This prevents food migration and therefore decreases inflammation.

In addition to having a role in gut integrity, white blood cells can also play a role in digestion. Oftentimes if someone has stomach acid or pancreatic enzyme deficiency, they will rely on their WBCs to digest their food. This is another way that WBCs get depleted and compromise the immune system. It is also important to note that over-exercise (long-distance running, etc.) can increase intestinal permeability and be a source of inflammation.

Exercise and Oxygen Delivery

Exercise can also improve circulation. This helps to deliver nutrients and oxygen to your cells and keep the healthy cells healthy. Breast cancer cells create a hypoxic environment that is associated with cancer progression. It is in the hypoxic environment that cancer thrives. The local conditions of tumor cell growth, known as the tumor microenvironment (TME), are characterized by low oxygen supply (hypoxia) caused by insufficient blood delivery. Hypoxic cancers have a strong invasive potential, increased tendency for metastasis, resistance to therapy, and a relatively poor clinical prognosis. Exercise increases oxygen delivery to tissues which may be one of the mechanisms by which exercise decreases breast cancer risk and progression. It is highly beneficial to increase our aerobic or our oxygen carrying capacity through exercise. This enhances the health of our cardiovascular system, which only serves to increase our circulation and oxygen delivery.

Exercise Regenerates the Mitochondria

In addition to being a metabolic disease, cancer is considered a mitochondrial disease. The mitochondria are the energy producing units of our cells. There are many environmental insults that damage our mitochondria and make us susceptible to developing breast cancer. Exercise increases mitochondrial function and promotes the repair and restoration process of our mitochondria. Exercise also increases the number and quality of our mitochondria which helps the body make more energy.

The research has revealed that exercise is found to reduce the risk and mortality of breast cancer, colon cancer, prostate cancer, endometrial cancer, ovarian cancer, and lung cancers. This is a key point here. Walking for only one hour per week at a moderate rate between two and three miles per hour will greatly assist your ability to maintain optimal health and healing. Walking for only one hour per week at a rate of two to three miles per hour was found to lower your risk of dying from breast cancer by 49%. Now these are astounding numbers! It just goes to show you that a little goes a very long way here.

Your Exercise Prescription

150 minutes a week of moderate intensity exercise (work up a sweat; you can talk, but you're breathy).

This Includes:

- Cardiovascular exercise
- Weight training
- Flexibility
- Balance

Five Basic Principles of Exercise Beginner to Advanced

1. Warm Up: five to ten minutes of an easy walk, bike or jog. Warming up prevents injury, muscle soreness and helps you feel looser during exercise. Warming up gradually increases your heart rate and prepares your body for higher levels of physical exertion.

2. Stretch: Takes about five to ten minutes and loosens up the muscles and ligaments. All stretching is done head to toe. Stretches should be held for ten to fifteen seconds while breathing into the muscles. Staying in tune with your body helps you feel into your stretch so you do not overdo it.

3. Exercise: Do something you enjoy for thirty to forty minutes. You should vary between cardiovascular and weight bearing exercise. Know that it all counts: you can use your own body weight, cables, dumbbells or bands. Begin slowly and increase your exercise routine gradually. You don't want to do too much too soon and risk injury or setback.

4. Cool Down: It is very important to cool down for five to ten minutes after you have exerted yourself with cardio and resistance training. Cooling the systems down tells the body it's time to slow down all the physiological functions like your heart rate, blood pressure, cardiac output, and metabolic activity.

5. Stretch Again: Stretching lightly after exercise helps you to prevent injury and keep your muscles and joints loose.

Some important points:

Do what you like and brings you joy. If you consider what you are doing stressful, it will put undue stress on your system and you will not achieve your desired result.

Do not exercise in excess of an hour. When you cross over an hour, this puts undue stress on your body and again will not serve your intended result which is to get and stay well! (I am talking about continuous exercise here, like running. If you are playing doubles or something that involves a lot of stops and starts, then just listen to your body.)

If you are over fifty, you need to prioritize weight training over cardiovascular exercise.

No exercising couch potatoes. Working out every day is great but you need to be active all day! Even if you have a desk job you can walk in between projects (we only have an attention span of ninety minutes max). Or be like me and get a treadmill and a standing desk. Our brains work better when we move.

Having a buddy makes it more social and more enjoyable. It also helps with accountability.

Make it a priority. Set time and make time. Put exercise on your calendar every day. The things we put in our calendar are the things that are important to us and the things that are going to get done. Make exercise and movement a priority.

If you are just beginning, set small achievable goals and let those goals grow. Healthy fitness and health goals build upon one another.

Most importantly, exercise preserves your body's ability to function properly. At the end of the day, if you don't move your body, you lose it. I know you are going through so much. There are going to be days where you just don't feel like it. There are going to be days that you are tired, busy, sore, in pain, uncomfortable, and all the other excuses we all make for not exercising. I want you to remember that small things matter. Even a little bit of exercise is beneficial. Exercise and movement are too important to your health to skip. And if you think something small can't make a difference, try sleeping with a mosquito in the room!

CHAPTER EIGHT - THE SECRET TO NOURISHING SLEEP

When I was a little girl, my Mom-Mom Ruth used to ask me three questions whenever I wasn't quite myself.

Bubuluh, are you hungry?

Do you need to poop?

Did you sleep?

Jewish grandmothers always know the questions to ask…without a moment of medical training she knew that children who are sick don't want to eat. She knew that not pooping caused big problems. And she knew that one poor night's sleep made you feel awful.

To this day, I still find so much value in these three simple questions and I use them frequently in my practice. In this chapter, we are going to focus on my grandmother's third question about sleep and explore why it matters so much on your journey to better health. We will discuss why sleep matters, the top reasons we don't get high quality sleep, why most Americans' sleep habits are artificial and processed, and what we can do about it. We will learn what happens when we sleep, and how to get the quality and quantity sleep that we need for true healing and repair.

Many of my patients that are currently going through breast cancer treatment or who are in remission tell me that they have difficulty falling asleep and staying asleep at night. They tell me that they can't seem to shut their brain off when they go to bed and even though they feel physically tired, they are mentally wired. Sometimes aches and pains or digestive troubles keep them from falling into a restful slumber and, as a result, their body never gets the time it needs to fully heal and repair. These are all very common issues and ones that we will address in this chapter.

Why Sleep Matters

It's no secret that sleep disorders are rampant in the United States today. Roughly seventy million Americans suffer from insomnia and twenty-two million suffer from sleep apnea per year. Anything less than seven hours of high-quality sleep per night can lead to serious health conditions such as heart disease, stroke, diabetes, and even cancer. Sleep deprivation has negative short-term ramifications as well as long-term such as obesity, low libido, depression, lowered immunity, and premature aging.

Sleep deprivation can also cause chronic inflammation. Even just one night of poor quality sleep can cause an elevation in inflammatory markers that can put you at greater risk for disease.

The timing of your sleep is important. Not only are we creatures of habit, but we are organisms that live by circadian rhythm, or the rhythm of the sun. We know that even if shift workers get adequate sleep they are still at increased risk of chronic disease. In a study of 1009 shift workers in Poland, the odds of developing breast cancer were twice as high in those that worked the night shift.[22]

The effects of poor sleep are almost immediate. You might notice that when you are sleep deprived you feel more irritable and make rash decisions. You may snap at your spouse or children without meaning to or feel trapped by the brain fog that you can't seem to clear. Your brain is inefficient, your memory is poor, and your temper is short. Strong sugar cravings are also another common side effect of sleep deprivation and studies show that sleep-deprived people eat around 385 excess calories per day!

---

[22] Szkiela, Marta et al. 2020. "Night Shift Work-A Risk Factor for Breast Cancer." International journal of environmental research and public health vol. 17,2 659. 20 Jan. 2020, doi:10.3390/ijerph17020659.

Conversely, when we get enough high-quality sleep every night our body goes into recovery mode and the benefits are numerous: improved immunity, more energy, increased problem-solving skills and clarity, decreased inflammation, weight loss, and overall better mental health. Sleep is also vitally important for cellular restoration, tissue growth, muscle repair, protein synthesis, and hormone regulation.

This is why it is imperative for you to get an adequate amount of restorative sleep at night to promote healing during your breast cancer journey. Sleep is where the healing happens!

The Reason We Don't Get Sleep is Because We Don't GET Sleep!

Lee and her husband spent their life in the wine business. During the day, Lee would man the store. They would come home at the end of the day, have dinner and her husband would go to sleep. This was Lee's time to work. She would work on her computer until about 2:00 in the morning, go to sleep, and get up the next day and do it all over again. This went on for forty years, until she was diagnosed with metastatic breast cancer.

In our fast-paced, Go! Go! Go! culture, sleep is oftentimes viewed as a sign of weakness and something only lazy, unambitious people do. As a society, we don't value sleep. Our society values the waking hours and the activity that happens during that time. I have heard many times from the many overachievers that surround me,

"I'll sleep when I'm dead."

Only when they are faced with their own death do they realize the stupidity of that plan. Many of us have a demanding lifestyle that we can't possibly keep up with and as we fall further and further behind on our seemingly never-ending to-do lists we too often sacrifice sleep to try to get ahead. If we're being honest though, skimping out on sleep or sleeping poorly at night actually has the opposite effect. In our efforts to get ahead, we actually fall further behind the often arbitrary goals, expectations, and deadlines we set for ourselves. Day after day we feel more fatigued, burned-out, sick, and fed up with the impossible standards we set for ourselves.

I like to say that we don't have a sleep crisis, we actually have an energy crisis!

In our society the average person over-consumes energy on a daily basis. We over-consume food that our body has to work on overdrive to digest, which compromises our ability to get restorative sleep at night. We over-consume oxygen by breathing too shallowly and too quickly, contributing to our chronic anxiety and stress. We over-consume information by watching too much TV (especially the news), spending hours upon hours on social media, checking our email, and responding to messages. This puts our brains on high alert at all times, making it difficult for us to get into a parasympathetic (rest and digest) state and fall asleep at night. Lastly, we over-consume light by staring at our computer or cell phone screen all day and then coming home from a long day at work only to stare at a TV or tablet screen. We also have bright overhead lights turned on all day that keep us awake and alert even in the evening when we should be starting to feel sleepy. All of these things are getting converted to more energy in our bodies and we are just not dissipating it. This is why so many people turn to artificial methods to help them fall asleep and stay asleep at night.

Most American's Sleep Is Artificial and Processed

Sleeping pills, alcohol, and marijuana—these are some of the most popular sedatives used in our country and they have terrible ramifications on our sleep cycle. These substances don't help us get restorative sleep and, in fact, actually disrupt our sleep! Studies show that chronic use of sleeping pills increases the risk of cancer more than smoking cigarettes. The whole concept of ingesting a substance with harmful side effects to try to help us fall asleep and stay asleep at night is part and parcel to the problem, because we're already taking in too much. Instead, we should be doing less and letting go of what no longer serves us.

Remember: Recreation does not equal rest and inebriation does not equal sleep!

There are also other things that can negatively affect your sleep at night. For example, drinking caffeine too late in the day can make you feel wired and anxious before bed, so if you are sensitive to caffeine or having difficulty falling asleep, I recommend limiting your caffeine intake to one cup of coffee or green tea early in the morning. Gluten and dairy can also disrupt your digestive system and make it difficult for you to get the deep, restorative sleep that you need. Lastly, I recommend fasting from all foods for at least two hours before you go to bed so that your body has enough time for proper digestion and so you won't be disturbed by acid reflux or indigestion while you're trying to sleep.

What Happens When You Sleep?

Despite the common perception that sleep is rest, sleep is actually an active process. When you sleep, you cycle through four key sleep phases multiple times per night. It is during this time that your tissues repair and your metabolism kicks into gear. It goes from digestion and fat storage to fat mobilization (as long as you do not eat before bed). Your immune system resets when you sleep, which is why sleep deprivation makes you more likely to get sick. Your brain processes what it encountered that day, deciding what to keep and what to purge. In addition, the lymphatic system of the brain, the glial system, gets rid of the waste and toxins that the brain encounters during the day. This is part of the reason why if you don't sleep well you have brain fog. Your brain is literally polluted! It is when you sleep that memories are sorted, and your hormones are regulated. Sleep is where your cellular repair mechanisms kick into gear.

Sleep cycles happen in 90-100 minute increments. If you interrupt a sleep cycle, you generally feel rather groggy. Sleep cycles are meant to be completed. This is why if you're hitting the snooze button every morning, you can ultimately feel worse than you would have if you just woke up because you are likely entering a new sleep cycle and waking up before you complete it.

When you prioritize sleep, you give your body ample time to process all the energy and food you consumed during the day. Your body then decides what information, experiences, food, and toxins need to be released. While you sleep, deep repair and regeneration is happening. In short, if you're not sleeping, you're not healing.

Remember: Sleep is not a luxury! Young to middle-aged adults need seven to nine hours of sleep every night, and seniors need seven to eight hours.

How Do You Get the Sleep You Need?

Like most things in life, sleep is a learned skill and one that needs to be cultivated. Most people don't know that there are things they can do right when they wake up in the morning and all throughout the day to help them sleep better at night. Below is the recipe for my best sleep hygiene tips for an amazingly therapeutic night of sleep.

- Get exposure to sunlight early in the morning, midday, and in the evening to signal to your body and mind what time of the day it is. Even just a few minutes several times a day will help reset your circadian rhythm! Try to carve out time to watch the sun rise and set and enjoy going outside for a midday stroll.

- Partake in joyful movement every day and try to do it as early in the day as possible. This will give you energy throughout the day and help you to feel sleepy at night. Do not exercise at night, as it will cause your cortisol (stress hormone) level to surge and prevent sleep as your body will think there is an ocean or a desert to cross.

- Limit caffeine, especially in the afternoon and evening. Caffeine can stay in your bloodstream for up to ten hours after you consume it, so it's important to minimize caffeinated beverages after noon if you are having trouble falling or staying asleep.

- Enjoy a low glycemic dinner in the evening and try to avoid all food within two hours of bedtime. Limit your water and tea intake after dark as well so that you aren't waking up to use the bathroom in the middle of the night.

- If needed, take 1-3 mg of melatonin at dinner time to help you fall asleep faster at night and stay asleep all night long.

- Limit your exposure to light, especially blue light, after the sun sets, as this can reduce your melatonin levels. I recommend wearing blue light blocking glasses in the evening. Try to turn off overhead lighting in your house in the evening and, if possible, replace your regular light bulbs with red bulbs as soon as the sun starts to go down. You can also use Himalayan salt rock lamps instead of turning on your overhead lighting. Lamps and low level lighting are preferred after dark.

- Invest in room darkening curtains or wear a sleep mask to block out light. We sleep far better in absolute darkness.

- Be sure to remove any electronics from your bedroom. Do not charge your devices on your nightstand or near your bed. Devices should be out of the bedroom when you sleep.

- Make sure your room is quiet or wear ear plugs.

- Tape your mouth before bed (one vertical piece of 3M tape) which will ensure nasal breathing and prevent snoring and sleep apnea.

- Turn off your WiFi at night and put your phone on airplane mode when not using it. Also, the less EMF stimulation you get during the day, the easier it will be to sleep at night.

- Make your bedroom a welcoming sleep environment and use it only for intimacy and sleep. Make sure your mattress, pillows, sheets, and comforter are all to your liking.

- Cool your bedroom to around sixty-five degrees Fahrenheit before bed. Our bodies need to cool down to sleep.

- Partake in soothing rituals before bed. Invest a few moments of your time journaling about your day and expressing gratitude. Carve out some time for peaceful meditation, or some rounds of breath work. Clearing your brain of clutter by doing a "brain dump" can also help relieve the mind racing that disrupts sleep.

• Enjoy a warm Epsom salt bath before bed while diffusing lavender essential oil to reduce aches and pains and promote relaxation. A warm bath will also allow the body to dispel heat and cool you for sleep.

• If you need to take a nap during the day, make sure that it's only for about ten to twenty minutes at most and that you do it before 5:00 p.m.

• Try to go to bed and wake up at the same time every day, even on weekends. I recommend being in bed ready to sleep by 10:00 p.m. and waking up at 6:00 a.m.

• If you're having difficulty sleeping, don't lay in bed trying to force yourself to fall asleep! Instead, turn on low light and read a book or try meditating.

I realize that you are not going to be able to do all of these things at once. Start with the basics and let the habits build. Make sleep a priority. When you do that, you will be rewarded with health. Be kind to yourself and aim for progress, not perfection. Remember, sleep is where the healing happens. If you are not sleeping, you are not healing.

CHAPTER NINE - THE HEALING MINDSET

Do you know what the number one predictor of how you will do through breast cancer and beyond is? It's how you think you'll do. Your mind, your perception of reality, is what dictates your health and your future. Your mind is both the most important thing and the one thing that you can surely control.

When you are facing a breast cancer diagnosis, the most important thing is to know that you will get well. Whatever you truly believe to be true will be true. My friend and colleague Chris Wark has an awesome quote in his book, Chris Beat Cancer. "Whether you believe you can do a thing or not, you are right." — Henry Ford

I want all of you to remember that everything is impossible, until someone does it. No matter where you are on your cancer journey, I believe that you can get well. Health can be achieved at any age and any stage, but it takes the right mindset.

We spoke in the beginning of this book about how breast cancer forms when the body is in stress chemistry. An environmental shift has taken place transforming you from the chemistry of joy to the chemistry of stress.

When we are in stress chemistry, our dominant hormone is cortisol. We actually only understand two basic states, danger or safety. When we are in danger, our body does what it has to do to escape said danger. This system worked great when we had a very limited amount of threats.

Nowadays, the things that threaten our safety are endless and boundless. Instead of actual threats, most of our stressors come as perceived threats. Our lives may be safe, but our jobs, our relationships, and our time is not. Our stress starts first thing in the morning with alarms, texts and calls. We listen to the horrors going on in the world on the news. We are polarized by the media outlets. We race to get to work, or the kids to school. We have deadlines, difficult relationships, financial pressures, not to mention the inescapable and impossible standard we are all held to with a seemingly perfect world displayed on social media. It's no wonder cancer rates are skyrocketing!

We are only meant to be in that sympathetic, fight or flight state for less than five percent of the time. Except with all that I mentioned above, today we spend almost equal time in a cortisol dominant state. Cortisol serves a great purpose when you need to run away from a tiger. Cortisol raises your blood pressure and your blood sugar. As glucose goes up, natural killer cell activity goes down. These are the immune cells that are responsible for controlling cancer. Cortisol directs your blood flow to the essential organs you need to run away from a saber-toothed tiger— your muscles and your heart. At the same time, it is diverting away from other organs, like your brain, your breasts, your gut, and your immune system. You don't need to think, digest, or detox if you are about to be eaten by a tiger. You don't need to protect yourself against the common cold if you are going to be consumed.

This system worked just fine then because if you escaped, you were safe for some time. Your body was allowed to heal. Plus, you metabolized all that cortisol when you ran from the tiger!

Today, there is no escaping the cortisol. Most of us are sitting at a desk, working in front of a screen. Maybe you are on book deadline (who, me?). Maybe you are creating it for yourself because you are a distance runner. Maybe you have a high-pressure job, or a difficult marriage, or your house is filled with teenagers. Whatever the constant stress is that's surrounding you, if you want to get well, you need to start building resilience now.

The Consequences of Stress for Me

It was March of 2018. I went to bed early because I had to be in the OR the following day. Something woke me at 2:15 a.m. I sat up, terrified. I had no sight in my right eye and my face was numb, like I had been to the dentist, only I hadn't. It took about thirty seconds for my sight to come back. The numbness remained. I didn't have any body weakness and being my typical workaholic, plow-through-it self, I went back to bed. After all, I had to be in the OR in the morning. I woke later that morning at my usual time, 5:45 a.m. My face was still numb. It remained that way all day. I was at the scrub sink outside of my OR and the surgeon next to me had a sister who was a neurologist. I confided in him what was happening and he summoned his sister. I finished my cases and had a work-up for what was threatening to be an MS diagnosis. Suffice to say that I was terrified.

I remember like yesterday what she said to me. She told me that the average person has symptoms for three years before they get an official MS diagnosis. While MS is an autoimmune disease, it is multifactorial. The one thing that everyone has as a trigger is STRESS. She instructed me that I had to get mine under control.

This, more than anything else, was the changing point for me. I had just one year prior been diagnosed with Graves' Disease. I was desperately trying to restore my health and now it was slipping even further away. There was only one place this road was leading and I didn't want to go there.

I don't want you to go there either.

Stress chemistry has a direct effect on our immune health. It weakens our immune system and it directly promotes tumor growth. Stress is linked with both the development and the progression of cancer.

What I want to map out for you in this chapter is how to get back to the chemistry of joy so that you can set the stage for wellness instead of disease.

There are many ways in which we can change our chemistry. It is important to have more than one tool in your toolbox to manage acute stress. At the same time, it is also necessary to look at your environment and eliminate the chronic stressors. We are talking about getting rid of unnecessary stress. Minimize your responsibilities, get rid of the " I have to's" that aren't really have to's. Choose to surround yourself with people who lift you up and do the things that bring you joy. Before you know it, you will be in a healing space!

In order to manage stress, you have to develop the skills. There are a multitude of things you can do to build resilience. Here are some:

- Meditation
- Breathing
- Gratitude
- Journaling
- Walking in Nature
- Exercise
- Tai Chi
- Qi Gong
- Massage
- Breathing
- Aroma therapy
- Art therapy

- Yoga
- Mind Based Stress Reduction
- Heart Math
- Essential Oils
- Bach Flower Remedies
- Spiritual or Religious Practice
- Emotional Freedom Technique (Tapping)
- EVOX
- MBSR (mind based stress reduction)
- Laughter

You have to be hiding beneath a rock somewhere for the last five years to not have heard about the power of meditation. Anyone who has had the privilege of attending a Dr. Joe Dispenza retreat has witnessed firsthand the power of what the mind can do. When I speak about the power of meditation, which I do often, I am met by this most frequent objection, "I can't clear my mind."

This is what is so wildly misunderstood about meditation. Let's dive deep into the power of meditation, gratitude, and more.

The Power of Meditation

Emily Fletcher was a Broadway actress who one day after having a panic attack on stage, set out for solutions. Through this, she discovered the power of mediation, practiced to master it, and then founded ZIVA Meditation. I learned of Emily when she was on Dr. Mark Hyman's

Podcast, The Doctor's Farmacy. Like most people, my objections to meditation, besides a general belief that mediation was for hippies and yogis, was that I wasn't capable of doing it. "I can't shut off my mind," I would say.

It was Emily that taught me (and hundreds of thousands of others) that you are not supposed to shut off your mind. The only time your mind stops thinking is when you are dead. That is the very thing we are trying to avoid in this book. What Emily so eloquently explained is that our mind is like a cocktail party and you are the hostess. Guests come in, you greet them, maybe you even spend a little time with them, but then you move on. You go back to being the hostess. You have to host your party and there are other guests. Some of them may be your husband's friends who you don't want to spend time with, so you say hello and move on. Or maybe it's someone you don't even like but invited out of obligation. You acknowledge them from across the room. Maybe the neighbor shows up uninvited and you tell them, "not today." Maybe you spot your best friend and you decide to sneak into the corner and spend some time with her. The thing is, you get to decide. You are the host!

Meditation is the same thing. Thoughts come into your head. You decide what stays or not. You decide what deserves time and what doesn't. You decide what to keep and what to discard. That is the power of meditation. You develop the power to control what you internalize. You keep what you want and discard the rest.

Meditation takes practice. It is a skill to be able to sit in a noisy room and hear nothing but the sound of your breath, to feel nothing but the seat beneath your bottom or the clothes on your body. We practice meditation for the many awesome benefits it has. Meditation reduces stress hormones, lowers inflammation and inflammatory markers, lowers blood pressure, helps to control pain, improves sleep, controls anxiety and promotes emotional health. It has also been clinically shown to reduce cortisol levels. The great thing about meditation is that it can be done anywhere. It is a very important skill to develop that will help you to reset your chemistry and better navigate your world.

Another invaluable technique that helps you to overcome transient stress is a controlled breathing practice. Many of us go through life taking small shallow breaths. When we are in a stressed state, we breathe rapidly, our heart beats rapidly, and we are very inefficient. All these mannerisms convey to the brain that we are in danger. However, by intentionally slowing our breathing, we signal to the brain that everything is safe. This can nip the stress response in the bud. There are many choices of breathing techniques to adopt. There is 4-7-8 breathing (in for four, hold for seven, out for eight, repeat that four times), box breathing, alternate nostril breathing, Wim Hof breathing, and many others. In fact, one of my favorite breathing exercises is a guided session with my friend Dr. Sachin Patel. Here is an interview he did with James Nestor, author of Breath.[23] How we breathe is of critical importance and making sure that you are breathing correctly and using your breath to manage stress is an awesome tool.

The Power of Gratitude

Next, we are talking about gratitude. When we are able to find gratitude, both in little and big things in our lives, it not only fundamentally changes how we feel about our lives, it fundamentally changes our chemistry. When we express gratitude, we are living in the moment with a deep appreciation for what we have. When we do that, we are actually able to see our world in a more positive light. Grateful people live longer and happier lives. A gratitude practice doesn't take much. Taking a few moments to jot down three things you are grateful for each day is all you need. If you ever have a day when things feel a little more difficult, you can refer back to your list and be reminded of all that's good. Grateful people find it easier to notice the positive aspects of life. Studies have consistently found that gratitude is positively related to well-being among breast cancer patients.

Qi Gong, or energy practice, helps to balance the electromagnetic energy of the body. It reduces fatigue, decreases cortisol levels, lowers

---

[23] Perfect Practice. 2022. "'You Will Never Breathe the Same Again' With Sachin Patel and James Nestor." https://www.youtube.com/watch?v=uB2QNiKNJ3o.

blood pressure, and increases your aerobic capacity. That's something that we want since cancer is an anaerobic process. By increasing our aerobic capacity we shift our chemistry. At the same time, exercise will improve strength, mobility, endurance, and our nervous system functions. Tai Chi will also decrease stress, anxiety, depression, improve your mood, your aerobic capacity, increase energy and stamina. It will improve flexibility, balance, agility, muscle strength and definition, and it helps you to live in the present. Anything you can do to create a positive mindset will improve symptoms of both breast cancer and breast cancer treatment.

Time for a Massage

Massage is another thing that can help us relieve stress and anxiety. It stimulates the flow of lymph, which promotes detoxification, balances your hormones, and actually increases your dopamine, which is your feel-good hormone. Massage increases the ability of your natural killer cells to to work, so it increases both the population and the strength of these cells.

Utilize Aroma Therapy

Aroma therapy is another great tool. Oils can be used to de-stress. They have the highest vibrational energy of any substance. They can help improve your immune function, as they tie together your brain to your immune system, they can help to reduce stress, anxiety, depression, and can help to alleviate pain and fatigue. There are many kinds of oils and oils are a very personal thing. The ones that are known to help with cancer are frankincense, lavender, rose, orange, pine, geranium, bergamot, lemon, and sandalwood.

Laugh — a Lot

Laughter truly is the best medicine. It boosts your immunity and improves your pain tolerance. It decreases the negative elements of the stress response. The funny thing is, it doesn't even have to be funny! You don't need a joke, you don't have to be laughing at anything. Laughter doesn't even have to be real. This is one of those times where you can trick your body into believing that something is happening that isn't. If you're laughing, it puts you into the chemistry of joy. That's why people say, if you're upset about something, just laugh, and it will change everything.

Practice Mindfulness

We all need to be more mindful. Mindfulness is a mental state that's achieved by focusing one's awareness on the present moment. It's not living in the past, not living in the future, but in the present moment, while calmly acknowledging and accepting one's feelings, thoughts, and bodily sensations, it's used as a therapeutic technique. The thing that we most use it for is STRESS!

Not All Stress is Bad

I want to be clear in saying that not all acute stress is bad. There are lots of stressors that are associated with things that are joyous, like planning a wedding. Marriage is a wonderful thing, but planning a wedding can be stressful. That kind of stress is okay. Having a baby is very stressful. It's also a wonderful, joyous event. The stress that is day in, day out, unrelenting, with no end to it, and no joy associated with it is the stuff that affects your health and puts you into stress chemistry leading to illness. So I want to ask you: where is your stress coming from? And the next question is. . . what are you going to do about it? Though some of us will be able to develop techniques that prevent us from internalizing the stress in such a way that it affects our chemistry, those of us that can't get there may have a situation that you have to get out of. You may need a different job. You may need to not work, you may need a different spouse, you may need different friends. You may have to say, "I'm just going to keep my distance from this family member or this situation for now because it's bad for me."

So, identifying and acknowledging where your stress is coming from is a really important part of your journey as stress impacts all aspects of your lifestyle and your physical health.

Cancer and Trauma

When I was trained, I was taught that trauma does not have a connection to breast cancer. I believe now that what they were referring to was direct trauma to the breast, like if you were to fall or get hit, or you were in a car accident and the seatbelt came across you and you got a bruise in your breast. In this instance, I agree there is no connection between direct physical trauma to the breast, which results in a bruise and the development of breast cancer later on.

However, significant physical and psychological trauma has lasting physiological effects on you. When we look at the breast cancer population in general, for people that are diagnosed with early breast cancer, stage one or two, about 35% of those people have trauma in their past. However, when we look at the metastatic population or the population of women that had breast cancer, and then had a recurrence, over 80% of them have unresolved trauma in their background. I want to stress the importance of finding some resolution to trauma. Your body, without question, is keeping score. Trauma can not be swallowed indefinitely. If you do not resolve past trauma, it will find a way of manifesting itself. You can't get it to go away, but you can give it a different meaning. You can give it a different interpretation, and you can find a way to stop it from continuing to hurt you.

There is ongoing research at institutions like Johns Hopkins where trained professionals guide women with metastatic breast cancer and a history of trauma through a facilitated journey using a medium like psilocybin. Psilocybin, more commonly known as magic mushrooms, allow the individual to experience the trauma in a controlled setting, only this time giving it a different meaning (that is where the facilitators come in). Then, with the aid of psilocybin, the new memory is hardwired in the brain. This gives the issue resolution and prevents the woman from reliving the trauma over and over again in the present. It is a way to safely put their trauma in the past so that they can move on with their lives. It's a way to stop hurting and start healing.

A diagnosis of breast cancer is also a trauma. It's normal to have very strong feelings in association with your cancer diagnosis. Anger, fear, resentment, sadness, and anxiety are all normal emotions for this diagnosis. It's important to deal with the feelings of sadness and fear, so that they don't become depression and anxiety. I want to stress that there is no expectation that your cancer diagnosis is going to make you happy. That's a ridiculous notion. However, there is a huge distinction between feeling sad, and being sad, or feeling depressed and being depressed. One describes a transient state, and the other an embodiment. There is an expectation when you get a cancer diagnosis, or any terminal diagnosis or bad news, that you should feel sad, and are transiently depressed. If that is what is coming up for you, it is important to feel that so that it does not become the embodiment of you. You should feel it and move on. The people that actually do the best following a breast cancer diagnosis are the people that are able to do exactly that. They're able to feel those feelings, but then they're able to move past those feelings.

Moving Forward

What are some of the emotions that have come up for you and all of this? What meaning are you giving to those emotions? Are they just contributing to stress chemistry? Are you able to find some meaning in your diagnosis, some meaning of the reason why you're in this position and how you're going to move forward in a positive meaningful way. Because if you're going to move forward in a meaningful way, then you need to learn from the past, but you can't live there. You need to get off and break away from the stress in whatever form that is not serving you.

We have direct clinical evidence that all of the above tools listed that aid with stress decrease cancer recurrences, lessen progression of disease, and lower blood sugar, blood pressure, inflammatory markers and medication use. They help you to cope with the side effects of conventional treatments, so that you can actually feel better and do better. They improve quality of life, and give you better emotional and physical health.

The key to any of these practices is doing them. Start by setting achievable goals and build habits. Once they become habits, you can increase the time and even the frequency. You can start with just five minutes of yoga in a chair and build from there.

Ultimately, the thing to remember is that the stress essentially isn't real. It's not something that's genetic; it's something that we can control. The stress itself isn't important. It's the meaning that we give to it that's important. As you can see, there are any number of different tools to help you manage your stress in your life. You don't have to have all the tools, but the more you have, the more resilient you will be. Not everything will work for everyone, but I want to be clear that I think that everyone should have some of these in their lives. There are so many things, so many ways to create a healing mindset and shift from the chemistry of stress to the chemistry of joy! What you need to do is build your toolbox with the things that resonate with you.

CHAPTER TEN - WTF IS EMF?

My mother-in-law, of blessed memory, was a brilliant woman. She was a member of MENSA, the largest and oldest high-IQ society in the world. She could speak to anyone of any age and engage them in captivating conversation. At eighty, she would talk about TikTok, fashion, music, and art — she literally couldn't have been more relevant. She was a true Renaissance woman. She spent her career as the general manager of the swankiest hotels in Miami Beach in the '50s, '60s and '70s. She was the Queen of Miami Beach and the seas parted for her wherever she went. She would entertain us for hours with stories about Sinatra, Dean Martin, Sammy Davis Jr., and the Rat Pack. She was amazing. What this smart woman couldn't figure out, though, is how not to keep her cell phone in her bra. When she died of pneumonia, she had a tumor in her breast just beneath where she kept that cell phone.

There are many things that cause inflammation and lead to disease. Many of them are obvious. It is easy to understand how processed food causes disease. It is easy to believe that chemicals like preservatives, pesticides, herbicides, and fungicides are bad for you. It's easy to see how bacteria, yeast, and mold make you sick. Unfortunately, there are many toxins that surround us that are completely invisible. They have no touch, no feel, no smell, and yet they are capable of tremendous damage. I am referring to the electromagnetic field.

I think we have well established the fact that chronic inflammation is the cause of nearly all disease. One of the greatest environmental toxins that causes inflammation is radiation. Here comes my public health warning: All wireless devices and anything with a plug emits radiation. I know that we don't always think about that. We have so many conveniences at our availability now, but we need to remember that all comes at a price. Every time you use a wireless device you are exposed to radiation. It's comparable to standing next to the microwave when it's cooking. Like the microwave cooks your food, your devices are cooking you.

Many of us rely on a system of trust where we believe that the EPA does rigorous testing and is there to protect us. The truth is safety guidelines were last updated in 1996. The current guidelines are based on short term exposure of radiation to five monkeys and eight rats. In fact, the NIH has recently halted these studies and says they do not plan to continue them, citing the technical challenges; in addition, the studies that were completed were on 2G and 3G devices, and now the majority of cell phones are 4G or 5G. (Which, by the way, emits an even greater amount of radiation.)[24]

Our modern world is surrounded by both an electrical and magnetic field that creates energy in the form of radiation. There are both natural and man-made forms of radiation, and these are known as the electromagnetic field, or EMFs. EMFs are a spectrum of electrical and magnetic wavelengths which are invisible to the human eye. These EMFs play a crucial role in creating light, facilitating communication through cellular phones, and powering various technologies but not all EMFs are equal regarding their impact on our health. EMFs create radiation. At times this energy is realized as sunlight. Other times the energy frequencies allow for cellular signals so that we can have phone communication. There are two broad categories of radiation: ionizing and non-ionizing. Ionizing radiation, like what is found in X-rays,

---

[24] Theodora, and Theodora. 2024. "EHT Op-Ed in the Hill: Why Is NIH Halting Research on Cell Phone Radiation Health Effects?" Environmental Health Trust - Education, Research, and Policy to Reduce Environmental Risks. (blog). March 4, 2024. https://ehtrust.org/the-hill-why-is-nih-halting-research-on-cell-phone-radiation-health-effects/.

mammograms, CT scans, bone scans, DEXA scans, and PET scans, are potent mid to high-frequency radiation that can destroy cellular health and damage DNA. Non-ionizing radiation is a lower frequency that historically has been claimed not to damage cells, and therefore was believed to be safe. This kind of radiation is what we find with cell phones, microwaves, Wi-Fi routers, bluetooth devices, home smart meters, computers, MRI machines, and power lines. For a long time, we considered non-ionizing radiation safe. However, we are now learning that just like low grade inflammation over time, lower frequency radiation is also dangerous.

We have known for decades the dangers of ionizing radiation. Ionizing radiation exposure has been linked to cancer. Mammograms cause thousands of breast cancers a year. CT scans make you five to ten times more likely to get cancer. This likely occurs due to direct DNA damage to the cells. In addition, radiation therapy, like what is used with breast cancer, can induce cardiovascular disease by damaging both the vessels and the muscle of the heart. This pro-inflammatory state leads to heart disease which is why women treated for breast cancer have two to three times the cardiovascular disease than their counterparts that weren't.

When it comes to low-grade EMF exposure, research shows that there is a detrimental effect on our immune system and mental health. The EMF causes sleep disturbance, and therefore makes you prone to a host of chronic diseases including obesity, heart disease, diabetes, anxiety, depression, autoimmune disease, and cancer.

In 2011, the World Health Organization (WHO) and the International Agency for Research on Cancer (IARC) classified radiofrequency electromagnetic fields as "possibly carcinogenic to humans," (Group 2B). It is in the same category as lead, DDT, and chloroform. Leading scientists argue it should be re-classified as a Class 1 "definite" carcinogen next to tobacco and asbestos. According to Nick Pineault, one of the world's experts on the dangers of the EMF, EMFs can cause dozens of health issues and lead to poor health and premature aging.

Devices that threaten our health include cell phones, cordless phones, tablets, laptops, gaming stations, microwaves, bluetooth headphones and wireless listening devices, fitness trackers, cellular smart watches, and smart meters in your home. The more of these devices that you have around, the more radiation you get. Radiation is additive and cumulative meaning that it comes in and stays in your body. Scientists link radiation to diseases, both long and short term. These diseases include cancer, infertility DNA damage, damage to unborn fetuses, sleep problems, memory and behavior problems, heart problems and many others. People have even become hypersensitive to radiation, where they can't even tolerate low levels of exposures, and they suffer during travel or while at home or work. EMFs can have a significant impact on your health, your job, and your social life. Sadly, the government is not going to protect you. You're going to have to do your own policing. You're going to have to do your own work in protecting you and your family from excess EMFs.

Protecting Yourself Against EMFs

Take a moment to think about all the devices around your home that are emitting electromagnetic radiation. The strength of the electromagnetic magnetic field decreases rapidly with increasing distance from its source. So you want to try to move yourself away from sources of EMFs as much as possible. Things like the microwave (which you should just get rid of by the way), your TV, your laptop, computers, touchscreens, tablets, your cell phone, your Wi Fi router, printer, any Bluetooth device, headphones, and XBox or gaming stations.

If you have ever had the rare privilege of trying to communicate with a teenager who has a device in their hand, you will know what I'm referring to. The EMFs emitted from these devices literally cause brain damage. Children who spend a significant amount of time on devices are cranky and miserable. That pretty much goes for adults too. I know that when I spend a considerable amount of time in front of a screen my head hurts and my vertigo gets triggered. There is no denying that the EMF has detrimental effects on the brain.

Another of the many ways that the EMF adversely affects our health is by affecting the health of our microbiome. This directly lowers our immunity, making us susceptible to a variety of illnesses. It can cause direct DNA damage. It can decrease melatonin production, which significantly decreases your body's ability to heal. It will increase inflammation because melatonin is our master anti-inflammatory hormone. It can disturb circadian rhythm, disturbing the quality and quantity of sleep. It decreases dopamine levels. Dopamine is our happy hormone, hence the cranky mood with EMF exposure. In doing all of that, it prevents you from doing what you're supposed to be doing. It interferes with achieving your best health.

Some of the symptoms of EMF toxicity are fatigue, ringing in the ears, insomnia, headache, dizziness, learning problems, heart problems, balance problems, leg cramps, eye problems, and more. I have become especially EMF sensitive, and I know immediately when I've had too much. I can't even ride in a car that has Wi-Fi. My head starts buzzing, I get a headache and become nauseated, and dizzy. We are all EMF sensitive, it's just a question of how sensitive you are.

Here is a plan for both decreasing your exposure and increasing your EMF detox!

- Move your router away from where you work.
- Decrease the amount of devices you have.
- Work with one or less devices around you.
- Remove devices from your bedroom.
- Track "indoor" time and increase your outdoor time.
- Decrease your blue light exposure (from devices).
- Wear blue light protective eyewear.
- Minimize device use after dark.
- Never eat in front of a screen as it disrupts the microbiome and your ability to digest and absorb nutrients.
- Open your windows whenever you can to help circulate the air and allow dispersion of radiation.
- Keep a safe distance of one foot from your devices.

- Work to decrease your screen time daily.
- Turn off your Wi-Fi when you don't need it.
- Put your Wi-Fi on a timer so that it is not on twenty-four hours a day.
- Put your cell phone in airplane mode when not in use, or better yet turn it off.
- Do not sit or work near a printer.
- Do not work with your computer on your lap.
- Unplug X-Boxes or gaming stations when not in use.
- Turn off hotspots in your car.
- Ground when you can (literally put your bare feet on the earth or invest in grounding shoes from Earth Runners or Rhizal).
- Take Epsom salt baths.
- Remove digital smart meters or put guards up around them.
- Stand on tin foil while brushing your teeth to discharge some of that day's radiation from your body.
- Sit on a grounding mat while working and sleep on a grounding mat at night.
- Do not screen for breast cancer with mammogram.
- Reserve CT scans for when absolutely necessary. Do not use them for screening.
- Do not use PET scans for screening.
- Do not use MRI for screening.
- Radiologic studies, with the exception of QT scan and ultrasound, should be done only when absolutely necessary.
- If you have to undergo a radiologic study, be sure to premedicate with the radiation protection protocol.[25]

---

[25] For more tips and resources, go to EWG.org or Nick Pineault's website: https://emfbook.com/.

CHAPTER ELEVEN - DETOXIFYING IN A TOXIC WORLD

We are unfortunately living in a sea of toxins. There are toxins in our food, our water, and our air. We're literally surrounded by substances and under near constant attack. There are heavy metals, stealth infections, fungicides, herbicides, plasticizers, fragrances and the like. Even our relationships can be toxic. All of this is wreaking havoc on our hormones and immune system. Toxins are everywhere and we can't possibly avoid them all, but there are things that we can do starting today to make things better.

From the very beginning, a baby born today will have over 250 chemicals in their cord blood. That only gets worse the minute they come out. Babies are barraged with plastic bottles, artificial nipples, infant formula, plastic pacifiers, detergents, sanitizers, and plasticized diapers. Toddlers are fed a steady diet of processed snack foods of grains, sugars, and inflammatory oils. Kids are slathered with toxic sunscreen. Teens are even worse. Scented shampoo, body wash, drug store lip gloss, shaving cream, acne treatment, birth control pills, lotions and potions are eating away at their hormonal health. As we progress into adulthood, things only get worse. . . more chemicals, more toxins, more stress, more disease.

Toxins are all around us. We need to understand where they are coming from, make every effort to reduce them, adopt some detoxification practices, and make a plan to do the best that we can. The best thing everyone can do is to create a daily routine which minimizes the amount of toxins that they use and maximizes detoxification.

Hiding in Plain Sight

Toxins are everywhere. They're in the water you drink. If you drink from plastic, they're there too. They're in the pans you cook your food in if you are cooking on a non-stick surface. They're in the cans from your favorite seltzer. They're in your plastic food storage or take out containers. They're in your toothpaste in the form of triclosan, an antimicrobial used to slow the growth of bacteria and fungus. There's fluoride in your drinking water and toothpaste which replaces the iodine in your thyroid hormone, rendering it ineffective. Dry clean your clothes? If you do, your skin is getting bathed in PERC. PERC is a reproductive toxicant, neurotoxicant, potential human carcinogen, and a persistent environmental pollutant. Furniture and clothing are treated with flame retardant, water repellant, and other things that lock in color. That is being readily absorbed by your skin. Like your Keurig or Nespresso? If you are using plastic pods, you are getting a daily dose of plastic with your morning cup.

Another area which needs attention is that of dentistry. Toxic substances used by mainstream dentistry have had a detrimental effect on our health. Beyond the fluoride treatments used by dentists, and the X-rays they repeatedly do, they are responsible for a considerable amount of chronic disease—including breast cancer. For decades, cavities were filled with metal amalgams. Dental amalgam is a dental filling material used to fill cavities caused by tooth decay. Dental amalgam is a mixture of metals, consisting of liquid (elemental) mercury and a powdered alloy composed of silver, tin, and copper. The mercury comprises 50% of the weight of the amalgam. As the amalgam ages, the mercury off-gasses as inorganic mercury and gets absorbed into the blood. According to the WHO (World Health Organization), exposure to mercury—even small amounts—may cause serious health problems. Mercury may have toxic effects on the nervous, digestive, and immune systems, lungs, kidneys, skin and eyes. Mercury is considered by WHO as one of the top ten chemicals or groups of chemicals of major public health concern. People are mainly exposed to methylmercury, an organic compound, when they eat fish and shellfish that contain the compound. People are mostly exposed to inorganic mercury from dental amalgams. Inorganic mercury is ten times more toxic than methylmercury.

The interaction between oral and systemic health are bidirectional and complex, involving many pathways. Much research on the inflammatory process and its relationship to oral and systemic disease is currently underway. However, we know that people with chronic oral infections are at risk for heart disease, inflammatory conditions and more. A recent study in Sweden stated that chronic periodontal disease indicated by missing molars seemed to be associated statistically with breast cancer. The conventional dental approach of drill and fill is creating disease decades later in the form of heavy metal toxicity and breast cancer.

Other areas of concern in dentistry are wisdom tooth extractions and root canals. When a root canal is performed it creates a devascularized cavity and sets the stage for chronic infection. For many women, this infection goes unnoticed as they do not create pain. Many of them are not even discovered until that woman is diagnosed with breast cancer. This is why I recommend that anyone with a history of a root canal have a cone CT of the mouth, read by a trained professional, to determine if there are any cavitations. With regard to breast cancer, teeth 2, 3, 14, and 15 are on the breast meridian. Studies have shown that breast cancers harbor the same bacteria found in these chronic infections in the mouth. I also believe that anyone with a diagnosis of breast cancer does the same thing. Remember to pre-medicate prior to your CT scan with the radiation protection protocol found in the resource section of this book.

If you have any metal amalgams in your mouth, or you have a history of root canals, I recommend working with a biologic or a holistic dentist to remove the toxins and improve the health of your mouth. I am currently working through this myself. I have discarded all my mainstream dental care and instead embraced Primal Life Organics

Dental Detox program to heal my gums and build my enamel. After only two weeks I already notice a huge improvement in the way my mouth looks and feels.

Marnie's Story

Marnie is a beautiful thirty-four-year-old woman who one day noticed a lump in her left breast. Her gynecologist thought it was nothing but asked her to have an ultrasound "just in case." A week later, Marnie had the experience no woman ever wants to have. The ultrasound tech who scanned her looked nervous and concerned. She excused herself from the room and returned moments later with the radiologist. The radiologist asked to do a biopsy as she was suspicious of breast cancer. The next day, the diagnosis was confirmed.

Marnie, prior to her breast cancer diagnosis, thought she was healthy. She was not overweight, exercised regularly, didn't drink out of plastic, minimized the products she used, prioritized sleep, was in a loving relationship, and preferred reading to mindless entertainment. Suffice to say, a breast cancer diagnosis was shocking to her!

Marni had a lumpectomy. Her cancer was aggressive and she was recommended to undergo chemotherapy, which she did. Just shortly after completing chemo, she noticed a mass again in the breast. Biopsy showed a recurrence.

This didn't make sense. It was too soon for the cancer to have come back. There must have been something driving it. This is when I started to work with her. She had four wisdom teeth extracted in her late teens and two root canals done. Her cone CT showed multiple cavitations in her mouth. She stopped chemo, and started on the path of reclaiming her oral health. Though the work took in excess of a couple months, it kept her cancer away more than any of the other "treatments" she had undergone previously.

Marnie's story is not unique. My friend and colleague, Dr. Veronique DeSaulniers, recounts her second bout with breast cancer in her book, Heal Breast Cancer Naturally, The Seven Essential Steps To Beating Breast Cancer. When she had her recurrence, she really struggled. She felt like an imposter. Not to mention that she was doing (almost) everything right. It was her decision to slow down a bit and embrace biologic dentistry that made all the difference for her. Her healing the second time around mostly involved healing her mouth.

The Dangers of Ethanol

Another major toxin in the world is Ethanol. This legalized drug has had a serious detrimental effect on our health. Everyone is aware of the chronic effects of heavy alcohol consumption including high blood pressure, heart disease, stroke, liver disease, and digestive problems. Heavy alcohol consumption can also result in cancer of the breast, mouth, throat, esophagus, voice box, liver, colon, and rectum. But what about small amounts of alcohol? For many years it was believed that small amounts of alcohol, like red wine, were beneficial. It turns out, that's not true. Even small amounts of alcohol can have health consequences. According to Dr. Tim Naimi, director of the University of Victoria's Canadian Institute for Substance Use Research, "Alcohol is harmful to the health starting at very low levels."

When you drink alcohol, your body metabolizes it into acetaldehyde, a chemical that is toxic to cells. Acetaldehyde both damages your DNA and prevents your body from repairing the damage. Damaged DNA sets the stage for cancer. At the same time, alcohol weakens the immune system, increasing the chances of getting sick or developing cancer. According to research by the American Cancer Society, alcohol contributes to more than 75,000 cases of cancer per year and nearly 19,000 cancer deaths. For some cancers, such as liver and colorectal, the risk exists only with excessive drinking. But for breast cancer, the risk increases with any alcohol consumption. According to the American Cancer Society, there is no safe amount of alcohol consumption for women. (don't shoot the messenger.) What I have landed on is this: There is no room for alcohol when you are actively cancering. What this means is that you are in treatment, within a year of treatment, or you are living with metastatic disease, you should not be drinking alcohol. Outside of that, if you want to enjoy a single, seldom cocktail or glass of wine, and you are otherwise in good health, then that is your choice. Just be sure that it is only a single and never on consecutive days.

The Problem with Mold Exposure

Mold is the next issue we need to tackle. Mold is ubiquitous! It's everywhere. For most people, that's not a problem. However, 25% of people lack the enzymes necessary to break down mold. These people become mold factories and the mold creates mycotoxins. It's these mycotoxins that are responsible for damaging your tissues. Because mold is so prevalent, I believe that everyone should check their home for mold and remediate if some is found. In addition, a HEPA air filter goes a long way in improving the quality of the air in your home. If you can't afford a whole house system, then an Air Doctor in your bedroom is a great solution. Most importantly, opening your windows and getting fresh air into your home is of the utmost importance.

Though I think it is beyond the scope of this book, I see a tremendous amount of mold illness in my breast cancer population. For many, it is one of the main drivers of their disease. Mold illness is a highly inflammatory condition. The symptoms of mold illness can be vague and varied. According to Dr. Todd Maderis, a mold expert, they include:

- **Psychiatric:** anxiety, fear, panic attacks, mood swings, irritability, anger, OCD, reduced ability to cope with stress, hallucinations, and suicidal thoughts
- **Cognitive:** decreased short-term memory, difficulty concentrating, difficulty learning new information, word-finding difficulty, reduced ability to plan and execute, lack of motivation, brain fog, and Alzheimer's dementia
- **Musculoskeletal:** muscle aches, sharp shooting pain, joint pain, morning stiffness
- **Cardiovascular:** palpitations, vasculitis, edema
- **Fatigue and chronic fatigue syndrome**
- **Respiratory:** shortness of breath, chronic cough, sinus congestion, nasal drip

- **Neurological:** headaches, migraines, tremors, vertigo, seizures, burning along the spine, sensitivity to light, sensitivity to touch, numbness and tingling, sense of internal vibration
- **Digestive:** abdominal pain, diarrhea, appetite swings, nausea, leaky gut syndrome
- **Eye tearing and itching**
- **Multiple chemical sensitivity (MCS) and EMF sensitivity**
- **Mast Cell Activation Syndrome (MCAS)**

If you suspect you have mold toxicity or mold illness, be sure to reach out to a trained specialist who can help you to recover. It will be nearly impossible to heal from breast cancer without resolving the mold illness.

Clean Water is Key

Water is another area that needs your attention. The amount of chemicals that are polluting our water is astounding. You need to know what is in your water. You can find out by going to the ewg.org/tapwater and entering your zip code. Ideally, you can filter for the chemicals in your water. The best system is an RO-reverse osmosis system. If you can only afford to do the sink in your kitchen, do that. If you can do a whole house system, even better. Even getting a Berkey Water Filtration System for drinking will go a long way toward decreasing your toxic load and improving your health. Another step would be to add an aqua sauna filter to your shower, so that you're showering with filtered water. And of course making sure that you're drinking out of glass or metal, no plastic bottles!

In the end, your goal is to reduce your toxic load. The way we do this is by decreasing the amount of toxins coming in and increasing the toxins you put out. Go through your home. What are you cleaning with? What are you washing your clothes with? Are you using dryer sheets? If you are, you are not only coating your clothes with toxic chemicals but you are also releasing those toxins in the air for you to breathe in. What do you wash your face with, your body, your hair? How do you moisturize your skin, your face? Do you wear makeup? Nail polish? The cosmetic industry is particularly full of ingredients that disrupt your hormonal system and your health. I realize that you can't change everything at once and no one expects you to. It's too daunting. What you can do is when you use up one thing, you replace it with something better. There are trusted brands like BeautyCounter or sites like CREDO that have product transparency. In addition, the EWG (Environmental Working Group) has a website where you can get a safety rating on a product or search for the safest option. So look in your closets, the kitchen, underneath the sink in the laundry room, in your bedroom, your bathroom, your car, and your office. Get rid of the chemicals, the fragrance, the perfumes, the plastics, the sanitizers,the antibiotics, the antibacterials, and all the other unnatural things that are adversely affecting your health.

The Dirty Dozen

We already discussed the importance of eating clean, real food. Get to know the Environmental Working Group's Dirty Dozen and Clean 15. You can find this right online at their website, ewg.org. The Dirty Dozen foods are things that you should only be consuming if they're organic. You should not consume the inorganic forms, as they are laden with chemicals. You can consume whatever conventional produce is available to you from the Clean 15.

Clean Up Your Cookware

Even the best quality food can become dangerous when it is not cooked or stored properly. This is why getting rid of nonstick pans and avoiding the microwave is so important. When you cook on a nonstick surface, tiny amounts of plastic are incorporated into your food. These plastics act as endocrine disruptors in your system and lead to cellular damage. So what you cook in and the method in which you cook matters. Investing in safe cookware goes a long way. Alternating between stainless steel, glass, ceramic, cast iron, and clay will both be safe and provide you with a variety of healthy minerals. Getting one good pan to cook in to start is probably all you need. (I have a number of suggestions on my website.) Food storage is another issue. If you store, or God forbid heat, your food in plastic, the plastic gets incorporated into your food. Going from cold to hot or hot to cold facilitates this process. You want to be sure that you're definitely never heating or freezing in plastic, and ideally it's best to not refrigerate in plastic. If you can store your food in stainless steel, glass or ceramic, that would be ideal.

The problem with plastic is that it acts as a xenoestrogen. Xenoestrogens are a family of compounds that compete for and act on the estrogen receptor on the cell. Though they dock onto the estrogen receptor, they are not estrogen. They overstimulate, they disrupt your normal hormonal balance, and eventually lead to cell damage. They directly cause cancer by both cellular damage and inhibiting your immune system. In addition to their direct cellular effects, they have to be detoxified by the liver, so they clog up your detoxification system at the same time, preventing it from doing the work it is supposed to be doing. Xenoestrogens include things like plastics, fragrance, the lining of aluminum cans, dishwashing liquid and laundry detergent pods, coffee pods, and disposable paper plates and cups. We are literally drowning in a sea of these xenoestrogens. I want to be clear that I am not talking about the estrogen that we're making in our body, but in fact, these synthetic estrogens, including birth control pills. They're hiding in places where you wouldn't think of. They are in your cosmetics, in nail polish, on cash register receipts, in baby toys, on your mattresses and pillows, toothpaste, antibiotics, hand sanitizers, air fresheners, scented candles, dryer sheets, pesticides, herbicides, fungicides, and many other materials commonly found in your home or office. Chemicals like triclosan, another xenoestrogen, is used as an antibiotic and it's embedded into all kinds of things so that they don't develop bacterial growth in them. They're in cutting boards and toothpaste and antibacterial soaps and cosmetics, cleaning supplies, and all of these places where you wouldn't expect them to be.

Forget Fluoride

Let's talk for a minute about fluoride. Fluoride is a byproduct of industry, and it actually has no benefit in terms of dental strength or health. It was put into dental products as a way to get rid of a toxic chemical. Fluoride that is stored in the body does so at the detriment of something. It displaces vital minerals, like iodine in thyroid hormone, therefore interfering with thyroid function. The amount of thyroid disease we have since adding fluoride to our water supply has exploded exponentially. It's mostly due to inactivity of the thyroid and fluoride directly interfering with thyroid hormone activity and function. In addition, fluoride ingestion can result in joint pain, stiffness, osteoporosis, muscle wasting, and neurological defects. For these reasons and more, I want to again express the importance of filtering your water for fluoride and not using fluoride toothpaste.

Makeup and More

Let's talk about our self-care routines. Believe me, I love products as much as the next person, but the average woman is exposed to over 150 chemicals in the morning before 9:00 a.m. We simply must decrease our toxic load. Think about what you actually need, instead of just randomly using all of these things.

Here are the top most common toxic ingredients that you want to avoid:
- Mineral oil
- Fragrance
- Diethanolamine, Triethanolamine, monoethanolamine
- Phthalates
- Propylene glycol
- Hydroquinone
- Triclosan
- Sodium lauryl sulfate
- Parabens
- Formaldehyde

- Petroleum
- Siloxanes
- Lead

Many cosmetics can contain heavy metals, talc, formaldehyde, mercury, phthalates, and methylene glycol. These things can be found even in expensive brands. We need to be really mindful about what we're putting in, on, and around us.

It is important to remember that anything that has a smell, good or bad, is toxic (with the exception of pure essential oils). There are many things that off-gas, like mattresses, pillows, furniture, new cars, carpet, stain guard, sealants, gasoline, synthetic clothing, dyes and coloring, paints and solvents. If you get a new car, make sure that you're opening your windows and improving ventilation. If you get a new mattress, try to see if you can allow it off gas somewhere for two weeks before you bring it into your home. Same thing with carpet—you want to avoid stain-guard and choose natural fibers. Open the windows for a few days in a newly carpeted area before moving in. Many of these chemicals are the gift that keeps on giving. They are forever chemicals. Once they take up residence in your body, they are very hard to get out. They are stored in places with an abundance of fat cells, like the breast, leading to disease. The breast, after all, is the canary in the coal mine. It is a very sensitive organ that is easily affected by toxins.

Clean Out Your Closet

Don't forget to look in your closet when searching for those toxic substances. The moisture wicking fabrics used to make athletic wear often contain PFAS. These forever chemicals are easily absorbed through the skin. An area of particular concern is yoga pants, underwear, sports bras, etc.

Vaginal Health

As vaginal health takes a particular hit with breast cancer and breast cancer treatment, I like to include it in our toxin discussion. The vagina is a very absorptive surface. You want to be especially careful of what comes into direct contact with it. This includes feminine products. Sanitary napkins and tampons must be unscented and organic.

Many of the vaginal lubricant products are extremely toxic. I like olive oil as a vaginal lubricant as it maintains the health of the vaginal microbiome. If you are looking for a commercial product, I recommend Julva. It was designed by my friend, Dr. Anna Cabeca. Better known as The Girlfriend Doctor, Dr. Anna is a triple board-certified physician and has dedicated her life to helping people age in the most gentle and healthy of ways.

Time to Detox

Once you have decreased the amount of toxins you are exposed to, it's time to detox. The first thing I have all of my patients do is a parasite cleanse every year. Parasites are ubiquitous. They are everywhere. Anyone who consumes raw food of any type is prone to parasites. In addition, in this hectic go go go world that we live in, we are all suffering from decreased immunity. This is the perfect recipe for parasite growth. You can find the link to my parasite cleanse in the Resources section of this book. If you do the cleanse and see a considerable amount of parasites (yes, you have to check your poop) then I recommend you do the parasite cleanse every six months rather than once a year.

Our body detoxifies through three main mechanisms. We rid our body of toxins through sweat, urine, and stool. This means that in order to detoxify we have to induce sweating, peeing, and pooping.

The sweating part is easy. You can either do that through exercise, steam, sauna, etc. One of my favorite therapies is infrared sauna. Unlike traditional saunas, which use heating systems to raise the temperature of the air within, infrared saunas heat your body while keeping the air around you at a constant temperature. As a result, your core temperature rises without the need to sit in a space that is 194 degrees Fahrenheit or higher. The hypothermic activity of infrared combats harmful cancer cells at the same time healing and regenerating our bodies at the cellular level. Hyperthermia is a known treatment for cancer. Infrared sauna can induce relative hyperthermia, which can help to clear cancer cells. Infrared is a great cancer treatment because it targets weaker cells while sparing good tissue from damage. Regularly using an infrared sauna improves blood circulation, which carries nourishment and oxygen to improve cellular health. This improves mitochondrial function, increases ATP production, and gives us more energy. It also helps deliver more oxygen to the tissues. This adds another anti-cancer effect as cancer cells cannot survive in highly oxygenated environments. All the while, you are ridding your body of toxins in your sweat. Be sure to shower immediately after your sauna to avoid reabsorbing the toxins. Infrared sauna generates a lot more sweat than other heating methods since infrared heat directly permeates the human body. People may spend more time in the sauna thanks to infrared heating, which makes it a better therapy. Infrared sauna is a wonderful way to help cleanse the body of PCBs, drug residues, acidic waste, and heavy metals. Infrared sauna can help to resolve the inflammation and edema and relieve stress,

As you can see, the benefits of infrared sauna are vast. In general, I like to layer therapies. Therefore, my recommendation is twenty minutes of exercise to induce sweating, followed by a cup of hot green or yarrow tea, and then into the sauna. Everyone's time in the sauna will vary. I aim to stay about ten minutes past the point that I'm uncomfortable. Regular use of infrared saunas can help detoxify the body, offer pain relief, improve sleep, give you better skin, promote relaxation, and improve circulation. I love my Sunlighten sauna as it is beautiful, comfortable, and has all the pre-set programs to give you the optimal dosages of far, mid, and near infrared light energy. The units now also have red light therapy which further stimulates the healing mechanisms of the healing mechanisms of the body. If a free-standing sauna is not in your budget, then I recommend a sauna blanket like the ones from Higher Dose. Both these products can be found in the resources section of this book.

Improving Lymphatic Circulation

Improving lymphatic circulation is also important. Your lymphatic system is primarily responsible for clearing toxins. The lymphatic system does not have any inherent pumping ability. Therefore, the only way to increase lymphatic flow is to do things that directly stimulate the lymphatics. This includes lymphatic massage, whole body exercises like rebounding, and manual lymphatic stimulation with dry brushing.

Rebounding, or jumping on a trampoline, increases white blood cells, stimulates your lymphatic system, helps to detoxify, boosts energy, and improves digestion. It can improve varicose veins, lead to weight loss, and prevent cancer by increasing lymphatic circulation and detoxification. It helps you to build bone mass and reduce cellulite. So get yourself a mini trampoline! There are so many great free programs on YouTube so get one and get started!

Oil Pulling

Oil pulling is another way to help your body to detoxify. It removes the toxins circulating in the bloodstream and the mouth. Just place a tablespoon of coconut oil in your mouth for ten to twenty minutes a day, swish it around, and then you spit it out in the trash afterwards. Make sure you spit it out in the trash, because otherwise it will clog your drain. This reduces inflammation and improves oral health.

Take a Detox Bath

Taking a detox salt bath using Epsom salts can be a wonderful way to detox at the end of the day. Combine a cup of Epsom salts with ten drops of lavender and a half a cup of baking soda to your hot bath water. This will increase sweating and improve detoxification. You can do this once a week as a detox therapy.

Castor Oil

Castor oil packs, placed either on your abdomen over your liver (right side of abdomen), or on your breast, are another great way to detox. All you need are the packs, castor oil, and a heating pad. I love the Queen of Thrones packs and do them myself several days a week. Castor oil packs pull toxins out of the liver and the breast through your skin.

Avoid Constipation

As I previously stated, we also clear toxins through urination and defecation. Making sure that you stay hydrated with clean water will help to flush your kidneys and eliminate toxins in your urine. Likewise, avoiding constipation is of vital importance. Everyone should be moving their bowels two to three times a day. If you are not doing that, you are not eliminating all the toxins coming in through the gastrointestinal tract. This means that they are being absorbed putting you at risk for a host of diseases including breast and colon cancer. There is a guide for avoiding constipation in the Resources section in the back of the book.

Detoxing with a Professional

All of the therapies we have spoken about thus far can be done on your own. However, there are some detoxification therapies that are best done with supervision, at least at first, but can be super helpful. Coffee enemas improve bile flow, increase the effectiveness of the body's own ability to bind toxins, and help to cleanse and heal the liver and colon. Until you master the technique yourself, it's best to seek some assistance.

Colonic irrigation or hydrotherapy is another detoxification therapy that also requires a professional. It can improve circulation, stimulate immune function, clear toxins and colonic debris, and help to boost energy.

There are also push/catch programs where you take a combination of herbs that help your liver to release toxins, and then they are caught up by toxin binding agents. These often require medical supervision.

Lastly, don't forget to look at the relationships in your life. Toxic relationships will have direct effects on your health. It's so nice when toxic people stop talking to you. Remember: that is a gift. It's like the trash took itself out.

I hope this chapter inspired you to take a gauge of your home and work environment, do a checkup, see what is there, do some testing, and see what you can improve. By no means do the above items represent every method of detoxification. However, this is certainly a great place to start. If you adopt these practices it will lead to a healthier you. Everything you do to decrease the toxins that go in and increase the toxins that go out will improve your health.

Here is your assignment:
- Eat real food.
- Buy organic when you can.
- Learn the Environmental Working Group's Dirty Dozen and Clean Fifteen.
- Throw away those nonstick cooking pans.
- Avoid high heat cooking (slow and low is the key).
- De-plasticize your home and your diet.
- Store your food in glass, metal or paper.
- Avoid fragrance.
- Look for the USDA Organic seal for your products.
- No hand sanitizers in your home except soap and water.
- Stop dry cleaning your clothes.
- Skip fluoride, make sure that you're filtering it out of your drinking water and don't use fluoride toothpaste.
- Pare down your beauty routine and remember that less is more.
- Replace your products one at a time with USDA certified organic brands. If you don't know where to start, start with lipstick and skin care because this is where we get the most exposure.
- Open your windows whenever possible to circulate the air.
- Make your own home cleaners. There are so many things you can just do naturally.
- Avoid antibiotics whenever you can.
- Use the Think Dirty app while you're shopping. It will give you a rating of 1-10 to tell you how "clean" or "dirty" a product is.

The less toxins you take in means the less work that your body needs to do to clear them. Happy hunting!

CHAPTER TWELVE - THE POWER OF CONNECTION AND PURPOSE

A breast cancer diagnosis can leave you with a myriad of feelings: fear, anger, betrayal, anxiety, nausea, pain, and devastation. These are all normal. All of these feelings are usually made worse by the conventional approach. Following a breast cancer diagnosis, women are generally whisked away into treatment. This sets the stage for feeling lonely, scared, and alone. I want you to know that you are not alone. I am here to tell you how you are already supported by reading this book. I want for you to dive into the power of my community, the power of that support, and others like it. There are many ways to find connection and support on your journey and it's important that you do.

We all need love and connection. Animals born in the wild and left alone will die. Babies born and have only their basic needs met, food and hygiene, do not survive. We are social creatures and need connection in order to thrive.

Surviving cancer is about so much more than treatment. Unfortunately, our system is focused on getting through treatment without giving any thought to the individual and what the rest of their life might look like. This is about much more than five-year survival. As previously stated, that is a minuscule amount of time for most women who get a breast cancer diagnosis. The goal is not merely to get people through treatment with little to no regard for long-term consequences.

The goal is to live a long, happy, healthy life. There are so many deficiencies in the current medical paradigm. One of the most glaring is the absence of the dietary and lifestyle inputs that contribute so much to health and well-being.

We don't need to look very far to see the power of social connection. The blue zones, those areas around the world where people survive well in excess of 100 years, are a shining example of the drivers of health. These people don't just live to be a hundred, they live well. They don't spend the last ten years of their lives hospitalized and debilitated. They are healthy. They are happy. They are productive and relevant. Of course, you can make an argument that there is very little processed food in their diet. That is true. There is also very little dairy in their diet. They grow much of their own food and therefore have very active lives. They mostly rely on their feet for transportation and that of course contributes to their overall fitness. However, perhaps the most important part of their societal arrangement is that their elders are an important and valued part of their society. They are as important to the success of their society as anyone. Their lives are full of purpose from the beginning until the end. When people need you, you stick around.

Breast cancer is not a blessing. However, that does not mean that nothing good can arise from it. I am a shining example of how a life-threatening disease can change you for the better. Had I not gotten sick, I'm certain that I would have never left surgery. I would have never found my way to you and this community. I would have never made the impact that I am making today.

Another example of this is my good friend Chris Wark. At twenty-six, when just starting out on adult life, Chris received a devastating diagnosis. Chris was diagnosed with stage III colon cancer. He knew little to nothing about the disease at the time of his diagnosis. Why would he? He was practically a child! This diagnosis would lead him on a path of self-discovery. He made some really difficult decisions and took a lot of criticism from his friends and family. I would love for you to listen to the Keeping Abreast with Dr. Jenn Podcast that we did together and to read his book, Chris Beat Cancer, to hear his whole story. Chris will tell you that while his experience was terrifying and awful, and I'm certain he wouldn't wish it on anyone else, it also led him to discover his life's purpose, create an invaluable community, and help hundreds of thousands of people heal from cancer. Chris will be the first to tell you that one of the main things that got him through was his deep connection to religion and God. Without that, he wouldn't have found the strength to do what he did. He made a lot of amazing changes and left the rest in God's loving hands.

Like Chris, I am a deeply religious person. We are taught in Judaism that God has put us all here on this earth with a unique purpose. My job in this world is to be the very best version of me and set out to accomplish what God put me here to accomplish. Your job in this world is to be the very best version of you and set out to accomplish what God meant for you to accomplish. My job isn't your job and your job isn't mine. I think we often feel as if what we do isn't enough. We compare ourselves to others and think,

"Wow, they're doing such great things."

Remember that whatever you do is great. We all bring equal value to the world and we are all equally important. The world needs everything in order to flourish.

The important thing here is to know that cancer is an opportunity. It's an opportunity to take stock of your life, figure out what's working and what's not, and ask if you are fulfilling your life's purpose. If you are not living connected, purposefully, and fully, then it's time to ask why? People who derive meaning from their diagnosis have a better quality of life and lower stress. We know that translates into reversal of disease, and also into longevity.

The Power of Connection

JJ Virgin, my mentor and health guru, talks about the concept of women living small. This fear of being big, of owning and occupying your space, creates internal strife. It creates the chemistry of stress. This is not what we are aiming to create. Being small leaves you lonesome, isolated and alone. It's time to break that pattern, own who you are, and step into your purpose. The world needs you to fulfill your purpose. You need you to fulfill your purpose.

Your community also has a significant effect on your health. According to Dr. Mark Hyman, the veritable figurehead of functional medicine, not only are positive relationships with others proven to improve our health and longevity, but they're also an essential resource in turning our dreams into reality. He says, "We can't do life alone."

Motivational speaker Jim Rohn tells us that, "You're the average of the five people you spend the most time with." He is also famous for saying, "Show me your friends and I'll show you your future."

Breast cancer can be an opportunity not only for you to improve your health, but for your friends and family to improve their health as well. When you heal yourself, it brings you joy. When you heal your community, it brings you elation. It has such a positive impact on your health and well-being. There is nothing more rewarding than being in the service of others.

Another example of the power of connection is pet ownership. Pet ownership is of great benefit to women with breast cancer. Pets not only bring us tremendous joy, but they give us purpose. Pet owners live longer and happier compared to those with breast cancer without pets. Pets can ease anxiety, decrease feelings of loneliness, improve symptoms of depression, reduce stress, improve physical health, and motivate you to stay active and alive.

Ultimately, the number one predictor of how long you will live is how strong your social connections are, and your desire and reason to live. It is so important to live a connected, meaningful life. It's what drives our existence. Living requires a reason to live, a raison d'être.

Susan's Story

Susan was a single mother of a toddler when she was first diagnosed with breast cancer. She told her doctor at the time of her diagnosis that all she wanted to do was live long enough to see her daughter graduate from high school. A few years after Susan's original diagnosis, she developed an in-breast recurrence. It was at this point that I inherited

Susan from my predecessor. Susan, in addition to having a large tumor in her left breast, also had shoulder pain. I sent her for a PET scan to look for metastatic disease and lo and behold she had bone mets. She again expressed her desire to live long enough to see her daughter graduate from high school. At the time, I did not know what I know now. I assured her that I would do everything I could to make sure that that happened. I look back on the years that I spent with her now with great regret. We set our sights too low. Susan lived an additional eight years and died the day after her daughter graduated from high school.

Our mind is such a powerful thing. I pray that this book empowers you to use the power of your mind to help you to maximize your health and your longevity. Set your sights high, be spiritually big, and soar through life.

Social support is the backbone on which all lifestyle changes will either succeed or fail. Changing lifelong habits can be really challenging, and you will need a strong support system. You need nourishing relationships. You need support to help foster healthy habits going forward. Community is everything.

Cancer, while not a blessing, can afford you the opportunity to reconnect with your loved ones, foster better relationships, prioritize your life, find a clear purpose, and give your life new meaning. This is all about you taking control of your health. You have way more power than you think. I know that when you unlearn that helplessness, you will realize all the power that you have within you. It's time to step into that power. You are all exceptional. I expect you all to be the exception.

Here is your homework for strengthening your social connections and building abundant health for your future:

- Take the trash out. Get rid of the relationships that are not serving you.
- Celebrate your wins with the people you love.
- Embrace spirituality.
- Find religion.
- Ask yourself what brings you joy and do more of that.

- Allow people to help you. You can't do this alone.
- Live big.
- Aim high.
- Believe that you are going to get well.
- Pay it forward and share what you are learning with your community.

CHAPTER THIRTEEN - SUPPLEMENTS, TREATMENTS AND OUTSIDE OF THE BOX APPROACHES

We are all biologically individual, so no two of our supplemental needs are going to be the same. What is right for one person is not necessarily right for another, highlighting our distinct biological needs. Remembering that food is medicine is crucial, as many nutrients we discuss should primarily come from food. However, given that our food is not as nutrient-dense as it used to be and many areas (especially in the US) suffer from soil depletion, it's important to focus on consuming organic foods.

Organic plants have the power to heal—because they are grown without chemicals, they develop more nutrient content to protect it from the sun, to heal when bugs nibble on them. Essentially, they are better equipped to survive and repair. And because they are healing themselves, when you eat them, they can also heal you.

We need to remain mindful of that. We want to get all our nutrients that we can from food because food is medicine. In this chapter, I am going to talk about specific nutrients that you can find in food and supplements alike.

Food Extracts

Let's start with food extracts. EGCG is a plant compound with antioxidant and anti-inflammatory effects. It comes from green tea, specifically matcha. (Matcha is ground-up green tea leaves.) When you drink matcha, you're actually consuming the whole plant. The benefits that you're getting from the EGCG in matcha are better than if you were just consuming EGCG because in the plant, the nutrients are synergistic. It's not just the one nutrient, it's all the nutrients in matcha. Matcha contains Vitamin C, selenium, zinc, magnesium, fiber, chromium and more.

When we supplement, it can be confusing to the body because there is too much single signaling. Our bodies know what to do with food far more than they know what to do with extracts. However, sometimes extracts may be necessary, like in the case of medicinal mushrooms, or, if you can't get it otherwise. In these instances, extracts can provide tremendous benefit. When food is a choice though, I always want you to choose food.

Broccoli Sprouts

Broccoli sprouts are a great example. There is broccoli sprout extract, which is really concentrated sulforaphane. But when you're eating broccoli sprouts, you're getting sulforaphane, and you're getting all the other components of the food. Again, your body knows what to do with food way better than it knows what to do with that individual extract. You mustn't take for granted the synergy that comes from getting nutrients from food. Yes, broccoli does have a lot of sulforaphane, but it also has a lot of Vitamin C and other nutrients.

Curcumin

In the cancer world, we talk about curcumin all of the time. There are many curcuminoids in turmeric. Instead of taking a curcumin supplement, you can consume turmeric root and get the spectrum of curcuminoids plus iron, magnesium, phosphorus, and potassium.

166

Brassicas

The brassicas, or the cruciferous vegetables, have DIM (diindolylmethane). Research shows DIM to:

- Prevent the effects of estrogen on cells
- Slow cancer cell growth
- Help with cellular metabolism and detoxification
- Boost antioxidants
- Promote weight loss
- Enhance memory
- Improve mood
- Reduce symptoms of PMS
- Promote muscle development

There is more than just DIM in the cruciferous vegetables. Crucifers are also rich in Vitamin C, folic acid, Vitamin A, iron, calcium, copper, selenium, and zinc.

Tocotrienols

Tocotrienols may reduce the risk of breast cancer by fighting free radical damage. Some studies also suggest that this form of vitamin E can slow the growth of cancer cells. A 2013 study found that tocotrienols could promote the death of breast cancer cells in the lab. Walnuts, almonds, hazelnuts, and macadamia nuts all contain tocotrienols, the Vitamin E's.

PUFAs

PUFA, polyunsaturated fatty acid, consumption is very important in maintaining balance in our inflammation/anti-inflammatory system. Eating two tablespoons of ground flax seeds every day is one way to achieve that. When you eat ground flax, you get the Omega-3s and so much more!

Garlic

Garlic is one of my favorite nutrients. It inhibits cancer growth, is an antioxidant, is antibacterial, antiviral, and has glucose and cholesterol lowering properties. Garlic contains high levels of potassium, phosphorus, zinc, and sulfur, moderate levels of selenium, calcium, magnesium, manganese, iron, and low levels of sodium, Vitamin A and C and B-complex. Garlic can be consumed raw or cooked, but not everyone does well with garlic. In this instance, the extract, allicin, can be consumed in the supplement form. I recommend allicin supplementation at the first signs of a cold or viral illness.

Blueberries

Blueberries are rich in anthocyanins. Blueberries have a ton of nutritional benefits beyond just the anthocyanins in them. They are rich in Vitamin K, which helps promote heart health. Vitamin K is also important in bone health and blood clotting. Blueberries are one of the best natural sources of antioxidants. They're thought to have the highest levels of antioxidants of any common fruit or vegetable. If you don't have access to wild, organic blueberries, then blueberry extract can be beneficial to you. Blueberry extract has been shown to exhibit anti-tumor activity against triple negative breast cancer cells and reduce their metastatic potential. Blueberries were shown to inhibit cell proliferation in triple negative cells with no effect on normal breast cells.

Mushrooms

All mushrooms have aromatase inhibiting properties. Instead of taking aromatase inhibitors, adding mushrooms to your diet every day can go a long way toward supporting hormone balance while protecting your health. These include white button mushrooms, oyster mushrooms, shiitake mushrooms, maitake mushrooms, and lion's mane. These are all culinary mushrooms. Most medicinal mushrooms, however, are non-culinary. You can get the benefit of mushrooms by consuming their extracts, like turkey tail and reishi.

Dietary strategies, emphasizing the consumption of whole foods rich in protective nutrients, alongside targeted supplementation, can offer an additional layer of support against cancer. These interventions aim not only to mitigate the toxic impacts of treatments like chemotherapy and radiation but also to empower the body's innate healing mechanisms.

Supplementing

The discussion around supplements is not just about counteracting treatment side effects but also about leveraging their potential to directly target cancer cells. Supplements such as apricot kernels, berberine, and high-dose melatonin, among others, have been identified for their specific anti-cancer properties. These substances, through various mechanisms, can inhibit cancer cell growth, induce apoptosis, and even target breast cancer stem cells, which are critical for preventing recurrence.

For those dealing with specific types of breast cancer, such as triple-negative or HER2 positive, the selection of supplements is fine-tuned to address the unique characteristics of these cancers. From DIM and melatonin to curcumin and specific phytonutrients, each supplement is chosen based on its ability to influence cancer pathways, stem cell behavior, or support the body's overall resistance to cancer growth.

When thinking about supplements and what your body might need as a supplement to your diet, you want to test and not guess. I routinely test several markers to help me decide what to supplement. Even if you have done the Nutrigenomics testing, it is important to test to see where you are functionally. All of these labs are common and readily available at any standard lab.

Here are the labs you'll want to order before you begin supplementing:

- CBC (a complete blood count): By knowing a blood count, you have information as to whether your white blood cells are adequate, which speaks to your immunity. Your red cell count and size speaks to adequate levels of iron, B12, copper and folate.

• B6, B9, B12: These levels speak to adequacy of the nutrients and can suggest methylation adequacy. Methylation is the process in which we create and metabolize hormones. Poor methylation can be a risk factor for breast cancer.

• Methylmalonic acid: Assesses Vitamin B12 sufficiency.

• Homocysteine (functional methylation assessment): Another marker of inflammation that lets us know how you're doing with methylation. It allows your clinician to put the B12, B9, B6 picture together for you.

• 25-OH Vitamin D: Vitamin D is the cornerstone of our immune system. Its function goes way beyond bone health. People with Vitamin D deficiency, of which there are a lot, have worse outcomes in cancer, with Covid and influenza, with chronic illness, with heart disease, and just about every chronic disease you could think of. You need to know your Vitamin D levels. Supplementation is based on your level, We are aiming for 60-100 ng/dL. For every 10 ng/dl you need to improve, you need 1000 IU of Vitamin D3. (Note, I never give D3 without K2.)

• hs-CRP: A high-sensitivity C-reactive protein is something that allows us to know how much inflammation is going on in your body, and whether or not we need to A) look for sources of inflammation and B) determine if you need more anti-inflammatory foods and supplements.

• ESR (erythrocyte sedimentation rate): Another marker of inflammation. This is more often seen elevated when we are talking about inflammatory conditions like autoimmunity and arthritis.

• Zinc and Selenium: We want to know your levels of zinc and selenium because they have a lot to do with your immunity, your thyroid function, your hormone balance, your blood sugar balance. Zinc and selenium are what I call

Goldilocks nutrients. There is a problem if there is too much or too little.

- Thyroid panel (including antibodies).
- Fasting glucose, insulin and A1C: Knowing your fasting glucose and insulin, and your hemoglobin A1C, is of utmost importance. Cancer is a metabolic disease. We need to know where you are in terms of your metabolic health and how to support your metabolic health. It is important to know whether or not you need berberine, Metformin, zinc and magnesium in addition to exercise to optimize your blood sugar levels.
- Iron and Ferritin: Too little iron is a problem but too much is inflammatory and promotes cancer growth.

The Key to Supplementing

Understanding the risk factors for breast cancer and the nutrients and foods that can support the body in this condition is crucial. For example, avoiding synthetic folic acid due to its potential to provoke cancer growth in certain genetic profiles and focusing on nutrients that support estrogen pathways and detoxification is essential.

Your supplement selection should be based on evidence and acquired from trusted sources to avoid contaminants and ensure efficacy. I think about supplementation according to where one is on their journey. Supplementation looks different if you're talking about prevention versus active treatment, recovering from treatment, or preventing recurrence. During active treatment, I often use a test called the RGCC, or the Greek test, to help guide my treatment decisions. This is a blood test that identifies circulating tumor cells and tests their sensitivity to a number of chemotherapeutic and natural agents. This test is available throughout the world but must be ordered by a certified provider. (If you are interested, you can find one on their website at https://rgcc-international.com/.)

Essential supplements during treatment include melatonin, selenium, folate from leafy greens, probiotics during chemotherapy and radiation,

Vitamin D, magnesium, turkey tail and reishi mushrooms, and Ashwagandha, among others.

Post-treatment supplements can help with recovery and combat the damage caused by the treatment itself. These include Coenzyme Q10, Omega-3 fatty acids, turmeric, and others, with specific considerations for their use during chemotherapy and radiation.

Specific supplements and pharmaceuticals have shown promise in targeting cancer cells and supporting the body through cancer treatment, such as apricot kernels (B17), berberine, high-dose melatonin, and more. Targeting breast cancer stem cells, supporting those with triple-negative breast cancer, and utilizing off-label pharmaceuticals can also play roles in a comprehensive cancer treatment and prevention strategy. When developing a highly individualized treatment plan, I use the RGCC to guide me. Remember: don't guess—test!

Protective nutrients are essential for shielding the body from the adverse effects of radiation and chemotherapy. Utilizing turmeric, resveratrol, Vitamin E, ginger, sulforaphane, and medicinal mushrooms like shiitake, maitake, and lion's mane, along with dietary inclusions such as green tea and and others like dandelion, milk thistle, cilantro, and parsley tea, can provide significant benefits. These can be incorporated into one's daily diet for their protective and health-promoting properties.

Radiation Protection Protocol

I highly recommend you use my radiation protection protocol that's found in the Resources section of this book. A radiation protection protocol emphasizes the importance of loading the body with antioxidants prior to exposure to ionizing radiation, such as mammograms, X-ray, PET, bone or CT scans, to mitigate the formation of free radicals. Recommendations include high doses of melatonin, liposomal Vitamin C, Vitamin D, the tocotrienols, and turmeric before and after exposure to radiation.

Gut Recovery Protocol

A gut recovery protocol post-antibiotic use, which often occurs with surgery or chemotherapy induced illness, focuses on special probiotics, nutrients for rebuilding the gut lining, and Vitamin D to restore gut health.

Breast Health

My breast health bundle includes modified citrus pectin (Pectasol), Vitamin D3 with K2, turkey tail and reishi mushrooms, magnesium, iodine, and liposomal melatonin. It is specifically curated to support breast health, can and should be taken indefinitely.

Antioxidant protocol

For those undergoing chemo, radiation, or surgery, a powerful antioxidant protocol is recommended to aid in recovery and combat cellular damage from chemotherapy and radiation. This protocol is vital for minimizing the long-term impact of treatment on the body. It includes probiotics, Vitamin D, fish oil, turmeric, pectasol, reishi, turkey tail, cordyceps, high-dose melatonin, and chlorella.

Supplementing During Treatment

Safe supplements during treatment aim to protect normal cells and include selenium, folate from leafy greens (emphasizing the importance of diet even during treatment), probiotics during chemotherapy to maintain gut health, and Vitamin D for its numerous health benefits.

Magnesium

Magnesium plays a crucial role in numerous bodily reactions and is especially vital during treatment. I consider magnesium an always supplement.

Mushrooms

Turkey tail and reishi mushrooms are also highlighted for their widespread use in cancer treatment protocols globally for their chemosensitizing properties and support against chemotherapy-induced fatigue, particularly in hormone receptor-positive breast cancers. In order to get the nutritional benefit of our mushrooms, they need to be heat-extracted. While there are some mushrooms you can cook and eat, turkey tail and reishi are quite bitter and are generally not consumed alone as food. These mushrooms are heat extracted, made into a broth, freeze dried, and sold as powders, capsules or tinctures. In this case, you will definitely want to consume them as supplements.

Melatonin

Melatonin, in combination with chemotherapy, has been shown to reduce the toxicity effects associated with treatment, indicating its importance during the treatment phase. Long term, it serves as a powerful antioxidant.

Mistletoe Therapy

Mistletoe therapy, derived from the European mistletoe plant (Viscum album), is used for its potential immune-modulating, cytotoxic, and quality-of-life improving effects. A strong advocate of this therapy, my friend and colleague, Dr. Nasha Winters, suggests that the use of mistletoe can help stimulate the body's immune system to fight cancer, improve the efficacy of conventional cancer treatments, mitigate the side effects of chemotherapy and radiation, and promote overall well-being.

Mistletoe is administered in several ways. It can be injected under the skin of the abdomen or the breast or used as an intravenous infusion. The method and dosage is tailored to your condition and needs. The exact mechanism by which mistletoe exerts its effects is not fully understood, but it is believed to contain several active compounds that can induce cancer cell apoptosis, inhibit angiogenesis (the formation of new blood vessels that supply tumors), and stimulate the immune system.

Dr. Winters emphasizes the importance of a personalized treatment plan for cancer patients, and considers mistletoe therapy as part of a broader integrative approach that includes dietary changes, nutritional

174

supplements, lifestyle modifications, and emotional support. She highlights the need for careful monitoring and coordination with a healthcare provider experienced in integrative oncology to maximize the benefits of mistletoe therapy and minimize potential risks.

Please note, while mistletoe therapy is widely used in Europe and has a growing interest in the United States among practitioners of integrative and naturopathic medicine, it is still considered an alternative treatment and should not replace conventional cancer therapies without thorough discussion with your healthcare provider.

Low Dose Naltrexone (LDN)

Another immune modulator is Low Dose Naltrexone (LDN). The FDA-approved drug naltrexone is typically used in higher doses to treat opioid and alcohol dependence. When used in low doses, LDN is believed to offer immunomodulating properties, making it of interest in the management of various autoimmune diseases, chronic pain conditions, and certain cancers, including breast cancer.

The proposed benefits of LDN for breast cancer patients revolve primarily around its potential to modulate the immune system. LDN is thought to temporarily block the opioid receptors in the brain, which in turn increases the production of endorphins and enkephalins—natural opioids that can boost immune function. This enhanced immune response might help the body recognize and destroy cancer cells more effectively.

Additionally, LDN is associated with anti-inflammatory effects, which can be beneficial since we know inflammation contributes to the development and progression of cancer. By reducing inflammation, LDN may help to create a less favorable environment for cancer cells to grow and spread.

Another potential benefit of LDN for breast cancer patients is its impact on quality of life. Some patients have reported improvements in pain management, mood, and overall well-being, which are significant factors in the treatment and recovery process for people with breast cancer.

It's important to note that while LDN shows promise, its use in cancer treatment, including breast cancer, is still considered experimental. More research is needed to fully understand its efficacy and optimal use in this context. I suggest you speak with your provider about exploring LDN as a complementary treatment. The low cost, minimal side effects, and potential benefits make LDN a really appealing option for those of you seeking adjunctive treatments for breast cancer, aimed at enhancing the immune response and improving quality of life.

Suggested List of Supplements

Below is a suggested list of supplements. Remember that in the functional medicine world we know there is no magic pill or single supplement that is going to "cure" you. We are interested in supporting your health and helping you to achieve optimal function.

Note that for those dealing with specific types of breast cancer, such as triple-negative or HER2 positive, the selection of supplements is fine-tuned to address the unique characteristics of these cancers. From DIM and melatonin to curcumin and specific phytonutrients, each supplement is chosen based on its ability to influence cancer pathways, stem cell behavior, or support the body's overall resistance to cancer growth.

The following is a list of supplements that are not only safe during treatment, but beneficial:

- **Selenium**: Serves to protect normal cells during chemotherapy and radiation.
- **Folate:** Found in all leafy greens.
- **Probiotics:** Help to support the immune system and gut health which can suffer during chemotherapy.
- **Vitamin D:** Central to immune health, Vitamin D levels have been directly linked to breast cancer outcomes.
- **Magnesium:** Magnesium is involved in over 300 reactions in the body and is paramount in regulating muscle and nerve function, blood sugar levels, blood pressure, brain health, and making protein, bone, and DNA.

- **Turkey Tail Mushroom:** Especially important with ER+ breast cancer.
- **Reishi Mushroom:** Especially important in HER2+ breast cancer.
- Ashwagandha: Works as a chemo-sensitizer while helping to alleviate chemo-induced fatigue. This is especially true for ER/PR+ breast cancer.
- **Melatonin:** Melatonin in conjunction with chemotherapy has shown reduction of chemotherapy toxicity such as cardiotoxicity (a major concern with some of the chemotherapy drugs prescribed for breast cancer) and renal toxicity. Melatonin has shown positive results in a number of clinical trials on patients with breast cancer. Used topically during radiation, melatonin can prevent the tissue damage associated with radiation.
- **Berberine:** Helps to lower blood sugar thereby lowering insulin levels and suppressing cancer growth.
- **High Dose Vitamin C (Ascorbic Acid):** Vitamin C given in high doses will generate hydrogen peroxide in the body. Normal cells are very efficient at clearing hydrogen peroxide but cancer cells are not. Therefore, cancer cells are readily destroyed by the hydrogen peroxide generated as a result of high dose Vitamin C where normal cells remain unharmed. Vitamin C in high doses also is a chemo/radiation sensitizer, making chemotherapy and radiation more effective. Note, you cannot get high doses with oral Vitamin C. If you are getting high dose Vitamin C infusions, you should avoid antioxidants like oral Vitamin C, alpha-lipoic acid, fish oil, glutathione, N-acetyl cysteine (NAC), Vitamin E, CoQ10, Sulforaphane supplements, Whey protein, L-cysteine or asparagus on the day of your infusion.
- Iodine: Iodine is essential to cellular health. Most people need to supplement as our diet has become extremely lacking in iodine.

Following the completion of treatment, there are several other supplements to consider that combat the damage caused by chemotherapy and radiation:

- **CoQ10:** Administered following breast cancer treatment, CoQ10 was found to reduce the markers of inflammation associated with cancer development.

- **Omega 3's:** These powerful anti-inflammatories reduce the inflammatory response. However, there is also evidence that they may increase response rates to chemotherapy. They are on the after list, but you should discuss with your doctor whether or not to include them DURING treatment.

- **Turmeric:** Though I encourage its use in cooking, the jury is still out as to whether or not it is helpful during chemotherapy. There are in vitro and animal studies that imply that turmeric may decrease the efficacy of certain chemotherapeutic drugs. The same is not true during radiation. During radiation, there is a substantial volume of evidence that curcumin is a radiosensitizer as well as a radioprotector of several normal tissues. Therefore, I recommend turmeric during radiation and beyond.

  - *A note about turmeric and tamoxifen: Because turmeric decreases the activity of the CYP3A4 enzyme, and this enzyme is the key activator of tamoxifen, turmeric is believed to decrease the effectiveness of that drug. The same is not true for the aromatase inhibitors. This only applies to tamoxifen.

- **Medicinal Mushrooms**
  - **Reishi:** Known as the mushroom of immortality. It is the queen of all mushrooms and has anti-cancer, anti-viral, anti-bacterial, anti-fungal and immune boosting properties. Also known to reduce stress, improve sleep, and lessen fatigue.

o **Turkey Tail:** It contains a variety of powerful antioxidants and other compounds that may help boost your immune system, increase natural killer cells, and fight cancer.

o **Super Immunity Blend:** Blend of medicinal mushrooms with five essential oils. Taken a minimum of 4x/day it is used to boost the body's immunity and cancer fighting ability.

o **Chaga:** for immunity, digestion, and skin health.

o **Cordyceps:** Known for energy boosting, it improves cardiovascular health, hastens recovery, and promotes healing.

o **Lions Mane:** The mushroom of the mind, helps to support brain function and aids in cognition, sleep, and mood.

o **Shiitake:** Is great for immune, liver, and cardiovascular health.

- **Pawpaw:** The major components of pawpaw are compounds known as acetogenins. They prevent the cell from making ATP, an important energy source. In lab studies, the extract killed cancer cells resistant to commonly used chemotherapy drugs such as adriamycin. I use pawpaw for people with chemoresistant disease, metastatic disease, or progressing disease along with other growth stopping methods. Paw Paw needs to be used in conjunction with your physician or provider.

- **VITAMIN D3:** Essential to the immune system, it reduces inflammation, inhibits cancer cell growth, inhibits the growth of blood vessels in cancer cells, induces cancer cell destruction. I always pair it with vitamin K2.

- **OMEGA 3 Fatty Acids**: Anti-inflammatory. Can be found in fatty fish and algae oil.

- **Melatonin:** The body's master anti-inflammatory hormone. Has potent anti-cancer properties. I prefer to use topical melatonin as it avoids having to go through the liver providing more reliable dosing. This can either be compounded for you at your local compounding pharmacy or you can make it at home by mixing a high-quality melatonin with your favorite organic moisturizer or carrier oil.

- **Vitamin C:** Low dose-oral: Boosts immune function and lowers inflammation.

- **High dose IVC:** can kill cancer cells and improve the efficacy of chemotherapy. If you are doing high dose Vitamin C, it is important to discontinue anti-oxidants, including oral Vitamin C.

- **Parent Essential Oils:** Oxygenates the cells and helps healthy cells heal.

- **Proteolytic Pancreatic Enzymes:** Taken between meals it strips cancer cells of its outer fibrin making them more vulnerable to treatments.

- **CoQ10 or Ubiquinol:** Powerful antioxidant, enhances the activity of some immune cells.

- **Quercetin:** Powerful antioxidant, anti-inflammatory, encourages cancer cell self-destruction, reduces cancer cell chemotherapy resistance. Can be consumed in small quantities daily as food.

- **Berberine, Alpha Lipoic Acid, and Chromium:** Help with blood sugar balance. Glucose is a primary food for most cancers, so blood sugar control is very important.

- **Bergamot:** Inhibits cancer stem cells. Not appropriate for those with low cholesterol. Must replace Coq10 with it.

- **Bee Propolis:** Appears to induce cell cycle arrest in breast cancer.

- **Modified Citrus Pectin:** Reduces metastatic potential by inhibiting galectin-3 which may block the "loss of anchorage" phase of metastasis. This can help prevent the cancer cells from traveling from the original site. I recommend the Pectasol brand.

• **Milk Thistle:** One study on the effects of silibinin on breast cancer cells concluded it inhibits the cells' growth and induces cancer cell death. Milk thistle may be "an effective adjuvant drug to produce a better chemo preventive response for breast cancer therapy."

• **Turmeric**: In breast cancer, curcumin, one of the active compounds in turmeric, inhibits cell proliferation, induces apoptosis, and acts as a potent antiangiogenic, anti-invasive, and anti-metastatic agent in vitro and in vivo.

• **Magnesium:** Used in over 300 reactions in the body, proper magnesium levels contribute to immune health, gut health, prevent constipation, increase bone health, brain health, and aid in sleep.

• **Ashwagandha**: Has been found to slow cancer cell growth, contribute to cancer cell death, and can be a chemo sensitizer. May also protect against chemotherapy induced fatigue. Useful in both hormone positive and triple negative disease.

• **Mistletoe:** Several studies have shown increased survival and reduction of chemotherapy causing side effects for breast cancer patients treated with mistletoe extracts. These are injections that must be prescribed by your provider.[26]

• **Ozone:** Studies show that ozone therapy can not only be used as a potential new chemotherapy but also utilized in combination with chemotherapy to enhance its efficacy. Ozone therapy has been used as medical treatment with the purpose of inducing apoptosis (tumor cell death), reducing tumor cell growth, inhibiting migration and invasion, and

---

[26] Marvibaigi, Mohsen, et. al. 2014. "Preclinical and Clinical Effects of Mistletoe Against Breast Cancer." BioMed Research International (Print) 2014 (January): 1–15. https://doi.org/10.1155/2014/785479.

reducing the formation of new blood vessels the tumor relies on.

When considering any or all of these supplements, it is important to work with your practitioner and decide what is best for you.

Off-label Pharmaceuticals Found To Enhance The Effects Of Chemo and Radiation (Especially With TNBC Or Chemo Resistant Disease)

- **Mebendazole:** An anthelmintic drug found to decrease tumor stem cell population and act as a chemo and radiation sensitizer. Pharmacologic option for resistant disease.
- **Doxycycline:** Inhibits cancer stem cells however not meant for long term use.
- **Niclosamide:** This is an antihelminthic drug used as a chemo and radiation sensitizer.
- **Claritin (Loratadine):** Found to inhibit the growth of tumors and promotes apoptotic cell death.
- **Tagamet (Cimetidine):** Works by the same mechanism to inhibit the growth of tumors and promotes apoptotic cell death.
- **Ivermectin:** May contribute to shrinking tumors in patients with triple negative breast.
- **Low Dose Naltrexone:** This has been shown to decrease recurrence and to help to reverse metastatic disease, especially in triple negative disease. Naltrexone in low doses can reduce tumor growth by interfering with cell signaling as well as by modifying the immune system.[27]
- **High Dose Statins:** When taken for short periods of time (pulsed) during cancer growth phases can deprive the

---

[27] Couto, Ricardo David, and Bruno José Dumêt Fernandes. 2021. "Low Doses Naltrexone: The Potential Benefit Effects for its Use in Patients with Cancer." Current Drug Research Reviews 13 (2): 86–89. https://doi.org/10.2174/2589977513666210127094222.

tumor cells of the cholesterol they need to build cell walls therefore "starving" them of a needed building block.

- **Pulsed NSAIDs (etodolac, celecoxib, diclofenac)**: Taken with a statin, NSAIDs will trigger apoptosis (cancer cell self-destruction). Best combined with low dose chemotherapy and high dose IV.
- **Vitamin C:** If still not responding, add glutathione lowering drugs (statins, feverfew, sulfasalazine, acetaminophen).
- **Anti-parasitic drugs with anticancer activity:** artesunate, ivermectin, albendazole.

Please note, use of any of the off-label drugs in this section for the purposes of treating cancer should only be done under the supervision of a physician capable of prescribing these drugs AND is familiar with their use in this instance.

This list is a partial representation of the supplements and pharmaceuticals that may be helpful for you along your breast cancer journey. It's crucial to consult with your healthcare provider before beginning any new supplement regimen, particularly if you are actively undergoing cancer treatment, to avoid potential interactions and ensure the supplements are appropriate for your specific health needs and treatment protocols.

There are several therapies that I refer to as "can't hurt, might help" therapies, that I included here in the supplement section. Though these aren't considered supplements, there are some outside of the box treatments that should be considered in your cancer healing plan. Things like ozone, hyperbaric oxygen treatment (HBOT), and RIFE therapy are treatment modalities that are helping to reverse cancer with no damage to normal cells. As such, I am hopeful that these treatments will become more accessible and available. Be sure to ask your provider about them and if you have the ability to access them, they would certainly benefit you.

Here's a closer look at how each of these therapies can play a role in a holistic breast cancer care plan:

Ozone Therapy: Ozone therapy is a remarkable tool against breast cancer. By introducing ozone into the body, either through blood ozonation or other methods, we can significantly enhance oxygen utilization by the body's tissues. This increased oxygenation helps to stimulate the immune system, fight infections, and may contribute to the reduction of tumor growth through improved cellular oxygen levels. Remember, cancer hates oxygen and struggles to survive in highly oxygenated environments. For women treating breast cancer, the enhanced detoxification and immune modulation offered by ozone therapy can be a valuable adjunct to their overall treatment plan, promoting a stronger, more resilient body environment less hospitable to cancer growth.

RIFE Therapy: I learned about RIFE therapy Dr. Kevin Conners of the Conners Clinic. RIFE utilizes specific frequencies to target and disrupt the viability of cancer cells, presenting a fascinating and non-invasive approach to complement existing treatments. The principle here is based on the concept that every cell, including cancer cells, has a unique electromagnetic signature. By identifying and applying the precise frequencies that resonate with breast cancer cells, we aim to weaken or destroy these cells without harming surrounding healthy tissue. While more research is needed to fully understand and optimize RIFE therapy for breast cancer, its potential for targeted action with minimal side effects makes it an intriguing option for integrated cancer care strategies. For more information on RIFE therapy, go to www.connersclinic.com.

Hyperbaric Oxygen Therapy (HBOT): HBOT is a powerful therapy that involves breathing pure oxygen in a pressurized environment. This process significantly increases the amount of oxygen your blood can carry, promoting healing and fighting infection. For women with breast cancer, HBOT offers multiple benefits. It can

184

enhance the efficacy of radiation therapy by making cancer cells more susceptible to radiation. Additionally, it supports wound healing and tissue repair, particularly important for those recovering from surgery or radiation-induced damage. Moreover, there's emerging evidence suggesting that the high-oxygen environment may create unfavorable conditions for cancer cells, potentially slowing their growth.

In integrating these therapies into a breast cancer treatment plan, it's crucial to do so under the guidance of professionals who understand both the conventional and alternative medical landscapes. Each woman's cancer journey is unique, and while ozone therapy, RIFE therapy, and HBOT hold promise, they should be considered as part of a broader, personalized treatment strategy designed to address your specific needs and circumstances. Always consult with your healthcare team to explore how supplements and therapies can best support your path to wellness.

Here's a quick reference guide to the supplements I recommend.

General Supplements for Breast Cancer Care:
- Vitamin D
- Magnesium
- Selenium
- Folate (preferably from leafy greens)
- Probiotics (especially during chemotherapy)
- Omega-3 Fatty Acids (fish oils)
- Coenzyme Q10 (CoQ10)
- Turmeric (Curcumin)
- Melatonin
- Ginseng
- Indole-3-carbinol
- DIM
- Sulforaphane
- Iodine

Specific Supplements for Treatment and Recovery

During Treatment:
- Selenium
- Probiotics
- Vitamin D
- Magnesium
- Melatonin
- Turkey Tail Mushroom
- Reishi Mushroom
- Ashwagandha (as a chemosensitizer)
- Ginseng
- High dose pancreatic enzymes
- High dose Vitamin C (during chemo)

Post-Treatment Recovery:
- C60 (Carbon 60)
- Coenzyme Q10
- Omega-3 Fatty Acids
- Turmeric
- Ginseng
- Immune Modulators and Adaptogens:
- Medicinal Mushrooms (Chaga, Turkey Tail, Agaricus, Lion's Mane, Shiitake, Cordyceps, Reishi)
- Ashwagandha
- Low Dose Naltrexone
- Mistletoe

Antioxidants and Nutrients for Radiation and Chemotherapy Support:
- Turmeric (Curcumin)
- Resveratrol
- Vitamin E
- Ginger Root

- Sulforaphane (found in broccoli sprouts, kale, cabbage)
- Medicinal Mushrooms (Shiitake, Maitake, Lion's Mane)
- Melatonin
- Chinese skullcap
- Ginseng
- Green Tea
- Dandelion Tea
- Milk Thistle Tea
- Cilantro and Parsley Tea

Supplements Targeting Specific Cancer Types:
- Triple Negative Breast Cancer: DIM, Melatonin, Vitamin D & K, Turmeric, EGCG, Fasting
- HER2 Positive Tumors: Tocotrienols (Vitamin E forms), Sorulen, Broccoli Sprouts, Curcumin, Olive Oil, Mistletoe, Beta Glucans, Fasting
- Pharmaceuticals with Off-Label Uses in Cancer Care:
- Mebendazole (anti-parasitic)
- Doxycycline
- Niclosamide (chemo and radiation sensitizer)
- Claritin (for high histamine levels)
- Tagamet
- Ivermectin (anti-parasitic with anti-cancer properties)
- Low Dose Naltrexone

I can't stress enough the importance of working with a qualified provider that can help you to navigate this wide landscape and safely coordinate any conventional treatment you might be undergoing with the modalities and possibilities mentioned in this chapter.

CHAPTER FOURTEEN - MENOPAUSE: DO WE HAVE TO SUFFER?

(The Controversy Over HRT After BrCA) Having come from a breast cancer family, and finishing my training in 2003 (the year that the Women's Health Initiative was halted), I came up believing that hormones were dangerous. Like many physicians that trained during my time, I was taught to believe that hormone replacement had no benefit and only risk. Therefore, it was to be reserved for women who absolutely positively couldn't live without it. Even in that instance, hormone replacement should be given in the smallest amount for the least amount of time. This is the belief system that I had for the first fifteen years of my practice. Like most people who come from breast cancer families or had a history of breast cancer, I believed that I was not a candidate for hormone replacement. When menopause hit me, I would just have to suffer through it. I remember my mother complaining for years about hot flashes and night sweats. As a society, we view the symptoms of menopause as trivial. They are something that we just have to deal with. Women are expected to white knuckle their way through this phase of life. In thinking this way, we have done women a terrible disservice and as a result women's health has suffered for decades. It's time to pull the curtain back and reveal the truth about hormones, the pivotal role they play in our health, and help women live their best lives—especially those women with a history of breast cancer!

For me, menopause was as bad as it gets. It started in the same way that most start: my periods became irregular. Unlike women who have the opportunity to skip cycles, my cycle instead came every three weeks. To say that my bleeding was heavy was an understatement. My periods were more like a horror film than anything else. The mood swings were intolerable. Everyone in my family knew what was happening. My husband would simply hand me the broomstick while humming the tune from The Wizard of Oz. When my periods stopped, there was some relief. However, the night sweats and hot flashes continued. They were joined by brain fog, dizziness, palpitations, weight gain, dry skin, joint aches, vaginal dryness, painful intercourse, uncontrollable crying, and a fuse that would go off so fast it would make your head spin. I did not go quietly into my good night.

I was so miserable. I knew that if I didn't do something I was going to get divorced. I was desperate and in search of answers. I knew HRT would relieve all of my symptoms but how could someone with my family history take hormones? Then one day it occurred to me that perhaps what I had been taught all these years might not be true. Maybe estrogen wasn't the villain it was being painted to be. After all, we have estrogen receptors everywhere in our body. Estrogen is basically the hormone of life and vitality. So if estrogen is the key to brain health, bone health, heart health, skin health, bone health, breast health, and reproductive health, how could it be bad? I felt compelled to look into the data. I found Avram Bluming's book, Estrogen Matters, and it saved my life. Now, I'm going to save yours.

Estrogen is one of the most controversial molecules that ever existed. We have taken to blaming estrogen for everything from PCOS to infertility to breast cancer. The belief that estrogen causes all these disease states is logical, widely accepted. . . and wrong. If estrogen causes breast cancer, it would mean that every woman was put on this earth for the purposes of getting breast cancer. If estrogen causes breast cancer, why do we see breast cancer exponentially more often during the time in our life when we have the least estrogen, when we are postmenopausal? If estrogen causes breast cancer, why don't we see it in teenagers, or pregnant women who have ten times the amount of circulating estrogen as non-pregnant women? If estrogen causes breast cancer, why are breast cancer rates increasing? We are modern beings living on an old gene code. Our genes haven't changed. Our estrogens haven't changed. Estrogen is not and has never been the problem.

I am using estrogen as a catch-all term. Truth be told, we have three types of estrogen in our bodies. E1, or estrone, is the predominant estrogen in the postmenopausal woman. Estrone is primarily produced by the adrenal glands. E2 is better known as estradiol. This is the strongest of estrogens and is made primarily by the ovaries of a premenopausal woman. E3, or estriol, is the predominant estrogen of pregnancy and made mostly by the placenta.

Our endogenous estrogens, those that we manufacture in our body, serve great purpose. There is a reason there are estrogen receptors in just about every tissue in the body. It's because those tissues require estrogen in order to be healthy. When a woman goes through menopause and there is a lack of estrogen in the body, all the tissues suffer. The deterioration of the body happens fairly rapidly in the absence of estrogen. Therefore, it is important to understand the functions of estrogen so that you can understand why you need it.

Here's why people have become confused. Approximately 70 to 80% of breast cancers are considered hormone positive. This has led to the false conclusion that hormones cause cancer. This misunderstanding is highly welcomed by the medical community because it aligns with their plan. The truth is that when we look at normal breast cells, they have hormone receptors on them. Having a cancer with hormone receptors on it means that they have preserved a portion of the normal anatomy of that cell. In some cases, we see an up-regulation, or an increase, of the number of hormone receptors on a breast cancer cell. This is a survival mechanism and in no way implies causation. If there is one thing that you take away from this book, I pray it is the understanding and knowledge that estrogen DOES NOT cause breast cancer.

The reason that this theory became so widely accepted is because the pharmaceutical industry invented estrogen blockers. It was both easy and convenient to blame cancer on estrogen because they created a drug for that. Had that not happened, I'm certain we would be having a very different conversation. Based on that false premise, an entire industry was created and women have been suffering ever since. Hormone blockade after breast cancer has led to a two-to-three-fold increase in heart disease in women treated for breast cancer along with increases in dementia, osteoporosis, arthritis, depression, anxiety, sleep disturbance, and an overall decreased quality of life. It's time to ask ourselves, "What are we doing?!"

It has been over twenty years since the Women's Health Initiative study was halted. A retraction has been printed. The authors readily admit that their conclusion that hormone replacement therapy causes breast cancer was premature, unsubstantiated, did not reach statistical significance, and was wrong. That said, it's hard to unring a bell. Decades of women, breast cancer or not, have suffered as a result of that study. It's time to unlearn that lie.

The pharmaceutical companies were anxious for hormone replacement to be wiped off the map. It had long been off patent. It was no longer a money-maker for them. Why give one substance that can help with all the problems when you can give seven medicines that might help with one? Instead of HRT, pharmaceutical companies could give SSRIs for depression, medicines for sleep, anxiolytics for anxiety, beta blockers for heart rate and blood pressure problems, statins for lipids, bisphosphonates for bone loss, acid blockers for reflux, NSAIDs for joint pain, and on and on it goes. When you think about it that way, it's easy to see the conundrum.

In the end, it begs the question: Does HRT cause breast cancer? If we look at the sixty-five studies done on hormone replacement therapy between 1975 and 2000, forty-five of them were estrogen alone replacement and twenty were combined hormone replacement therapy. In the estrogen alone group, 80% of the studies showed no increased risk, 13% showed a slightly increased risk and 5% showed a decreased risk in breast cancer. In the combined HRT studies 80% showed no increased risk, 10% showed a slight increased risk, and 10% showed a decreased risk. Not exactly damning evidence for hormone replacement. Quite the opposite.

In 2003 with the "stop the presses" release of the findings of the WHI, several things happened. Overnight, three million women stopped their hormone use. Physicians stopped prescribing hormone replacement. And what happened with breast cancer incidence? Well I'll tell you what didn't happen. It didn't go down. Breast cancer incidence steadily climbed despite less and less HRT use. It's not your hormones, ladies! Environment—yes. Xenoestrogens—check. Radiating women over and over again with mammograms—absolutely. But not HRT. Estrogen doesn't cause breast cancer.

The case against HRT is a bad one. We are way overdue in dispelling this lie. HRT does not cause breast cancer.

The question now becomes: what about after breast cancer? Does hormone replacement make you more likely to have a recurrence? The data says no. There have been many studies looking at hormone replacement in the breast cancer population. Though the numbers are small, with the exception of one study the outcomes were all favorable in support of HRT after breast cancer.

Studies have suggested that hormone replacement therapy may reduce the risk of recurrence and death in postmenopausal women who have undergone breast cancer treatment. Additionally, some studies have found that hormone replacement therapy reduces side effects associated with chemotherapy and radiation therapy, such as hot flashes and fatigue.[28]

What was that one study that was the outlier? The HABITS Study. The HABITS study (Hormone Replacement After Breast Cancer Is It Safe?) was one of two Swedish trials looking at hormone replacement in the breast cancer population. Like the WHI, the HABITS study was also halted prematurely based on non-statistical significance. The study was halted after only two years due to what they believed was an increased

---

[28]Pfeifer SM, Taplin SH, Flockhart DA, et al. Effect of Hormone Replacement Therapy on Breast Cancer Recurrence in Postmenopausal Women: A Systematic Review. J Natl Cancer Inst. 2008;100(8):564-573. doi:10.1093/jnci/djn0873.

incidence of breast cancer recurrence in the HRT group. It is important to note several things about that study. The first Is that there was no difference in the groups in terms of lymph node positivity or distant disease. Those that recurred in the HRT group did not develop advanced disease any more than the ones that didn't take HRT did. Local recurrence is meaningless in the scheme of things as it does not impact survival. Next, only the group that got combined hormone replacement had an increased risk of recurrence. The estrogen only group actually had a decreased risk of recurrence. Finally, the only group that was at increased risk of recurrence was the group that took both tamoxifen and HRT. Though we will never know the answer for sure, what I suspect is that too much synthetic estrogen is ultimately going to lead to problems. Tamoxifen, after all, is a synthetic estrogen and a known carcinogen.

At the end of the day the decision as to whether or not to use hormone replacement is ultimately yours. The evidence that bioidentical hormone replacement is good for your health is indisputable. BHRT when started within ten years of menopause (the earlier the better) leads to better heart health, brain health, gut health, skin health, bone health, lung health, vaginal health, bladder health, better blood pressure, blood sugar, improved mood, less anxiety and depression, more energy, and a better outlook on life. If you have completed cancer treatment, or even if you are living with disease, BHRT, done in the context of all the other health promoting habits discussed in this book, can make you healthier and thus decrease your risk of a whole spectrum of diseases including breast cancer. As my friend Dr. Anna Cabeca famously says, "Menopause is mandatory but suffering is optional."

Please, don't suffer.

If you are looking for someone to help you with hormone replacement, look no further than the Dr. Heather Hirsch Collaborative. Dr. Heather is expanding her practice throughout the US and can help you safely navigate this landscape.

CHAPTER FIFTEEN - WHAT'S NEXT: TESTING, FOLLOW UP, AND CONCLUDING THOUGHTS

I have said repeatedly through this book that we don't guess, we test. It's time to talk about what those tests are.

Depending on where you are in your journey will dictate what tests you have and need. If you are just starting out, I recommend getting an initial lab panel which includes looking at a blood count, lipids, electrolytes, kidney and liver function, markers of inflammation, key nutrients, hormones including a full thyroid panel, tumor markers, and markers of metabolic health. You can view my initial lab order and ideal values in my resources guide on page 207.

You will need your healthcare practitioner to order these labs for you and help you to understand the results.

Initially, with my own patients, I am looking at gut health, immune health, nutritional health, and metabolic health. I am also doing some genetic testing to see what their genetic susceptibilities are. (This is not to be confused with genetic testing that is routinely done looking for gene mutations.) I am testing for nuanced information to determine how to support my patients' heart health, hormonal health, brain health, and detoxification pathways. I am always looking at the whole person and how to provide long term support. Health is a marathon, not a sprint.

If you have invasive cancer and evidence of lymph node disease, I like to order a circulating tumor cell test. I generally work with RGCC, but there is a company called DATAR that also measures circulating tumor cells and circulating cancer stem cells, and then provides you with both chemotherapeutic and natural agents that they are sensitive to. This test can be extremely helpful in knowing who needs treatment, and which treatments are most effective for you.

I am not a fan of CT scans, PET scans, or bone scans as they deliver a significant amount of ionizing radiation, and have a threshold of approximately 0.5 cm, which is 500,000 cells. I do not recommend them for initial staging or follow up as I prefer to follow laboratory markers of health.

Following treatment, I generally recommend surveillance including lab work and safe imaging modalities if desired. The following is my plan for going forward.

What I don't recommend

Mammogram: A mammogram is an X-ray of the breast that can detect masses or abnormalities that may be cancerous and represent recurrence. It can detect non-cancerous lesions too, like calcifications due to fat necrosis. Mammograms can directly damage the tissue with ionizing radiation and put you at greater risk of recurrence. I do not use mammograms to screen for cancer as I don't believe in using a test that causes cancer to screen for cancer. In my opinion, mammograms should never be used to screen a healthy, asymptomatic person for cancer. If you are going to have this study, please follow my radiation protection protocol included in the resource section of this book.

MRI: An MRI uses magnetic fields and radio waves to create detailed images of the breast tissue. This can help detect small tumors or areas of recurrence that may not be visible on a mammogram or ultrasound. MRI requires gadolinium as a contrast medium. Gadolinium is a heavy metal and does accumulate in the body. Anything that is stored in the body is done so at the expense of something we want and need. For this reason, MRI imaging should be reserved for necessity only. MRIs are notorious for false positive findings, meaning that they call attention to many things that are not of clinical significance. I do not use MRI anymore for screening or surveillance because the gadolinium is a problem. If you decide to undergo an MRI, please take 60 mg of zinc one to two hours prior to your study to prevent absorption of gadolinium, and continue for the next three days. The MRI protection protocol can be found in the resources section of this book.

CT Scans/Pet Scans/Bone Scans: CT scans, PET scans and bone scans use ionizing radiation to create 3D reconstructions of the body. These all deliver a much higher dose of radiation than mammograms and therefore should be used only when absolutely necessary. I don't believe in using imaging to survey for metastases or distant disease. Studies have not shown a survival benefit to follow up imaging and each time you have one of these studies you INCREASE your risk of recurrence. If you are going to have any of these studies, please follow my radiation protection protocol found in the resources section.

The following is what I do recommend:

Self-Breast Exam: Whether screening or post treatment, I believe in self-breast exams. No one is going to know you better than you know yourself. Breast examination should be done once a month. This should include a visual exam followed by palpation. The most sensitive part of your hand is your fingertips. To examine your breast, use your fingertips to go around your breast in a radial fashion starting outside and running your hands over the surface of your breast toward your nipple. A mass in the breast feels like a bump in the road. If you have undergone radiation, the texture of your breast does change. However, most people will still recognize a change when it happens. Once a recurrence reaches a certain size, it can often be felt while examining the breast. Don't forget to look at your breast noticing changes in size, shape, and texture. There are also instances when breast cancer recurs in the skin so please examine your skin when you examine your breast looking for white or pink firm painless nodules.

Ultrasound: An ultrasound uses sound waves to create images of the breast tissue. This can help identify a mass, determine whether it is a fluid-filled cyst (which is almost always non-cancerous or benign) or a solid mass. In general, every cancer is a solid mass but not every solid mass is cancer. Ultrasound is fairly non-specific so if something is seen on ultrasound, it will likely require another study or a biopsy for clarification.

Biopsy: A biopsy involves taking a small sample of tissue from the breast or the skin of the breast and examining it under a microscope to determine if it is cancerous. This would be used if a new mass was detected and found to be suspicious for cancer. With a needle biopsy, the standard of care is to leave a small metallic clip behind as part of the procedure. If you do not want a clip, you need to state that in advance.

QT Imaging: This is novel technology that is non-radiating, painless, fast, inexpensive, and has forty times more resolution than MRI. It requires no contrast, no compression, and call backs are extremely rare. This FDA-cleared technology is the only imaging modality with functional capability. This means that if a mass is detected, you can return in sixty days and a doubling time can be determined. Cancer cells have a doubling time of less than 100 days and lesions that are benign or very slow growing have a greater doubling time. Knowing the doubling time prevents unnecessary biopsies, over-diagnosis, and over treatment. This imaging modality will forever change the way that we screen for breast cancer and I am making sure that it is readily available over the next few years all across the United States. It will replace mammograms and MRI both for screening and follow up purposes. It will also be used to determine how well treatments are working and if and when people need further treatment.

Lab Work: This is my preferred method of follow up. Following metabolic health, Vitamin D levels, tumor markers, markers of inflammation, functional testing, and circulating tumor cells. These are the least invasive, radiation free, and reliable methods of determining ongoing health. Remember, at the end of the day, BREAST HEALTH IS HEALTH!

CONCLUSION

Breast cancer confuses us. The reason why we're so confused is because we think of breast cancer as breast cancer. I hope this book has helped you to discover that's not exactly true. Breast cancer is so many things. As we have learned in this book, breast cancer is trauma. Breast cancer is divorce. Breast cancer is mouth infections, mold illness, or heavy metal burden. Breast cancer is any number of things that adversely affect our body and prevent it from doing what it is supposed to do. We were created by God as perfect machines. Unfortunately, we live in a very imperfect world. But there is hope. That hope is YOU!

I pray that you have found this book to be informative, useful, and inspiring. It is important to understand your diagnosis. It is equally as important to understand that the solution to all of this lies within you! Breast cancer is not an accident or bad luck. You're having breast cancer doesn't mean that you have a bad breast. Breast cancer is a normal response to an abnormal environment.

To thrive through breast cancer, you must first decide that you want to live. Think about the reasons you want to live, write them down, and remind yourself of them every day. Make plans for your future. Commit to radical changes in your life and be prepared to take action. Health is not something you can inherit or purchase. Health needs to be earned. It only comes to those that take total responsibility for their health.

When you are ready, ask yourself why you think you got breast cancer. Many people know. They know that they had a very difficult year or two prior to their diagnosis. A divorce, a move, a job loss, a death in the family, being a full-time caretaker, financial worries, a trauma, a viral illness, mold exposure, a prolonged infection, chronic stress, a series of vaccinations, poor gut or dental health, any of these can adversely affect your immunity and allow for breast cancer to happen. In addition, we are literally living in a toxic soup filled with chemicals that are sabotaging our health and setting the stage for cancer. Asking these questions is not to provoke blame or shame, it is to empower you to take your control back. You have so much more power than you think!

Set out on your path to create your anti-inflammatory life. Remember, inflammation is the root of all disease. If you have a breast cancer diagnosis, and your proverbial sink is overflowing with toxins, you're going to need to mop up the floor. Sometimes conventional medicine is just that. But remember, it's just a quick fix and a band aid. Unless you turn off the faucet, unless you get rid of whatever is triggering your illness, the next manifestation of your inflammation is just waiting around the corner. The path to health starts now with everything you have learned in this book.

If you are one of the lucky ones able to see the message in your diagnosis, then perhaps you can transform your life into something with even more meaning and purpose. At the end of the day, know this. There is no change without change. We can't get better in the same environment that we got sick. Transformation requires transformation. I hope that you now have the information you need to enact positive changes in your environment and your health so that you can lead a healthier and more fulfilling life than ever before. I pray this book empowers you to be the change you need and the hero of your story.

If this book was enough to get you on your path to health, great. If you need more, visit us at realhealthmd.com.

If you want to keep up with me, listen to my weekly podcast, Keeping Abreast With Dr. Jenn. You can find it wherever you find your podcasts.

If you are wondering about QT Imaging, visit perfeQTionimaging.com.

Thank you for sharing this time with me. This was a labor of love, and I am honored and privileged to share it with you.

With Love and Gratitude,

Dr. Jenn

ACKNOWLEDGEMENTS

As I sit here and reflect on the last thirty years, it's hard to believe that this is my life. I have enjoyed such tremendous privilege. Though it has come as the result of tremendous work and some considerable hardship, the rewards of my work have been unimaginable. There is no greater privilege than helping someone heal from breast cancer. To be a pivotal part of someone's health makes my heart soar.

My aunt, Jill, wrote an article about me when I was eleven saying that I was going to be a doctor. What a forecast that was. Having been an unfocused child, no one, myself included, saw this coming.

To my parents, who are extremely proud, the best thing you ever did was doubt me. It made me strive even harder for success.

I have so many people to thank for making this book possible, starting with my aunt Jill. She has spent her career as an accomplished writer and had originally agreed to write this book for me. She then decided that it would not be authentic unless I wrote it myself. She was right. Had she followed through, I would have never had this experience and so for that and all of her love and support, I am grateful.

To my brilliant sister, Tracy, who painstakingly went through this manuscript to help find all the mistakes no one else did. You always were the writer in the family. I love you and I am so grateful for your help and your gift.

My team has been absolutely amazing through this process. They somehow gave me the time and space to write this book while seamlessly running my practice and supporting me where I needed it. Stephanie and Rachael, I am so grateful to you and all that you do to make my life possible. Thank you.

My fellow authors know the commitment of writing a book. Having written every single word of this myself, this represents a year's worth of nights and weekends and time away from my family. Albert, you are my biggest fan and my greatest supporter. You have given me everything I ever wanted. I cherish our marriage, our children, and grandchildren. I would be nothing without you. Thank you for giving me the time and space to hit this milestone. While I can't promise you I won't write another book, I can promise that it won't be anytime soon. I look forward to making up for time lost and to creating some really special memories together, starting tomorrow.

To my boys Andrew and Will, I pray that someday you look back with tremendous pride on how hard your mom worked to change the world. I wasn't there for everything but I tried to be there for the important things. I am extremely proud of the gentleman that you are morphing into and I believe that having a hard-working mom played some role in that.

I have been inspired by so many people in my journey as a surgeon, then a patient, and now as a holistic physician. In no particular order, I want to thank my cousin Linda Creed whose life inspired me to want to challenge the world of breast cancer. I want to thank Dr. Diana Dixon-Witmer and Dr. Dahlia Sataloff for taking me under their wing and showing me how to be a surgeon and a lady. I want to thank Dr. Gordon Schwartz of blessed memory, and Dr. Anne Rosenberg for training me to be the best surgeon I could be. I want to thank Dr. Mark Hyman for opening my eyes to functional medicine and Dr. Liz Boham for showing me what it really means to be a great doctor. I want to thank Dr. Sachin Patel and JJ Virgin for their hours of mentoring, brilliant advice, and for opening the doors of possibility for me. To the ladies that fluffed my feathers and told me to fly, I couldn't be more grateful. You gave me courage, advice, inspiration, constructive criticism, and most of all were shining examples of what is possible. Thank you Lauren Powers, Cynthia Thurlow, Dr. Kellyann Petrucci, Dr. Nasha Winters, and Dr. Veronique Desaulniers. Without your example, I could never be the author, podcast host, Summit host, and leader that I am. I want to thank Dr. Thomas Lodi, my brother from another mother, for the hours of awesome conversation. What you've done amazes me and I strive to be a better doctor because of you. I want to thank Dr. John Klock for bringing me into his world and helping me to write the next chapter of my life. This is going to be a big one!

To Lisa G., Lauren K., Patti S., Laura G., Amy H., and Gevura D., you are the best friends a girl could ask for. I am in awe of all of you and all that you do. Your love and support carries me. You are the wind beneath my wings.

And with that, I'll say,

Bye for now!

RESOURCES

The following are resources I mentioned throughout the book.

To access the most up to date resources, protocols, and products, visit: https://drjennsimmons.myflodesk.com/thesmartwomansguideto breastcancer or scan the QR code below.

Any items referenced below and in via my website are things that I personally use. However, I have no control over the quality or consistency of any of these products and have no direct relationship with the companies referenced. This resource section is intended for informational purposes only and should not be construed as a guarantee or endorsement of any product or service mentioned. Any claims made about the products or services are based on the information provided by the manufacturer or service provider and should be verified with them directly. Individual results may vary, and any reliance you place on the information provided is at your own risk. Additionally, please note that this section may contain affiliate links, which means that we may receive a commission if you make a purchase through those links. Your support is greatly appreciated and helps us continue to provide valuable content. Thank you for your understanding!

Dr. Lodi's Juice Fast

Yields 2 quarts of juice depending on the freshness, ripeness, and water content of the vegetables. Drink up to 4 liters a day for 2-3 weeks.

Ingredients (organic)
10 stalks of celery
2 cucumbers
2 bunches of kale
2 bunches of spinach
1 lemon
1/4 - 1" piece of fresh ginger root
1 granny smith apple
7-10 stalks of parsley (add last)

Instructions:

- Please substitute any ingredient that does not taste good to you or is unavailable for you. Keep in mind, I recommend including cucumbers and celery (for water volume) and at least one brassica vegetable.
- It is always helpful when the juice tastes good to you. When conducting a proper juice fast, small amounts of fructose (sugar from fruit) do not present major harm. Therefore, if you need to make it a little sweeter initially, do so, but decrease as you get beyond day three.
- Buy enough ingredients for a week's worth of juices.
- Store with FreshPaper* or to extend the life of your fruits and vegetables. Portion the vegetables out according to the number of juices you will make (i.e., enough veggies for 3-4 qts of juice per day for a week, then portion pack veggies in 7 bags). Pack bags with green veggies. Note that cucumbers, lemons, apples, and ginger are prepared at time of juicing.

- When you bring the vegetables home, cut off the root end of spinach and celery to separate. Wash immediately. When possible, use of 3-6% hydrogen peroxide to clean vegetables and neutralize petrochemicals and insecticides. You can add ½ cup of 3% hydrogen peroxide to water and cover vegetables. Let soak for 20 minutes. Residual hydrogen peroxide in low concentrations remaining on the vegetables does not present any harm.

- Use a salad spinner to dry spinach and kale. Place all other vegetables on towels to air dry thoroughly. If using paper towels to dry and store veggies, use the chlorine-free variety. Remember to insert a FreshPaper* sheet to the container.

- Use an auger juicer (AKA: masticating juicer) or a hydraulic cold press juicer.

- Add each ingredient to the juicer separately, making sure to leave the parsley for last because parsley tends to bind in the juicer.

- The juice will normally last up to 48 hours. For the juice to retain maximum enzyme and nutritional content, drink your fresh juice immediately or at least within the first 4-6 hours after being prepared. It is important to drink your fresh pressed juices within 24 hours.

- If you are going to work, juice the amount you will need and store in airtight mason jars leaving as little air at the top as possible. Store in the refrigerator upon your arrival.

- If juices cannot be consumed quickly, freezing will preserve many nutrients and enzymes (just be sure, in this case, to leave ample room at the top of the jar for the juice to expand when frozen or the jar will break).

- Drink a minimum of three quarts per day, although 3-4 quarts is best when doing a juice fast.

- The goal should be to juice fast for 10+ days without any other meals. But, if you cannot, even shorter durations of juicing provides benefits.

Additional Notes

- Continue taking your prescribed medications while on your juice fast.
- Avoid caffeine and do not consume any alcoholic beverages.
- Juicing includes high concentrations of bioavailable nutrients delivered to the cells that are lining the digestive tract.
- Juicing allows for a relative reprieve from the work of digestion, hence an opportunity to heal.

Real Health MD's Guide to Safe Supplements During Treatment

Making the decision to undergo chemotherapy and radiation is never an easy one, as they are carcinogens (cancer causing) themselves. If you have weighed the benefits and the risks, and made the decision, we want to make sure that you are doing the most for yourself throughout the process. There are ways to eat, drink, move, think, and supplement during treatment that not only improve the efficacy of treatment but also help to guard against the harmful side effects. The following is a list of supplements that are not only safe during treatment, but beneficial to use during treatment. Dosing of these supplements can vary from individual to individual and product to product. I recommend using reputable brands from pharmaceutical grade suppliers and manufacturers. Do not purchase your supplements from the grocery store, the drug store, or Amazon.

- **Selenium:** Serves to protect normal cells during chemotherapy and radiation.
- **Folate:** Found in all leafy greens.
- **Probiotics:** Help to support the immune system and gut health, which can suffer during chemotherapy.
- **Vitamin D:** Central to immune health, Vitamin D levels have been directly linked to breast cancer outcomes.
- **Magnesium:** Involved in over 300 reactions in the body and is paramount in regulating muscle and nerve function, blood sugar levels, blood pressure, brain health, and making protein, bone, and DNA.
- **Turkey Tail Mushroom:** Especially important with ER+ breast cancer.
- **Reishi Mushroom:** Especially important in HER2+ breast cancer.
- **Ashwagandha:** Works as a chemo-sensitizer while helping to alleviate chemo-induced fatigue. This is especially true for ER/PR+ breast cancer.

- **Melatonin:** Melatonin in conjunction with chemotherapy has shown reduction of chemotherapy toxicity such as cardiotoxicity (a major concern with some of the chemotherapy drugs prescribed for breast cancer) and renal toxicity. Melatonin has shown positive results in several clinical trials in patients with breast cancer.

- **Berberine:** Helps to lower blood sugar, thereby lowering insulin levels and suppressing cancer growth.

- **High Dose Vitamin C (Ascorbic Acid)**: Vitamin C given in high doses will generate hydrogen peroxide in the body. Normal cells are very efficient at clearing hydrogen peroxide, but cancer cells cannot. Therefore, cancer cells are readily destroyed by the hydrogen peroxide generated as a result of high dose Vitamin C where normal cells remain unharmed. Vitamin C in high doses also is a chemo/radiation sensitizer, making chemotherapy and radiation more effective. Note, you cannot get high doses with oral Vitamin C. If you are getting high dose Vitamin C infusions, you should avoid antioxidants like oral Vitamin C, alpha-lipoic acid, fish oil, glutathione, N-acetyl cysteine (NAC), Vitamin E, CoQ10, Sulforaphane supplements, Whey protein, L-cysteine or asparagus. High dose Vitamin C is anything over 10 grams, however ideal dosing is more on the order of 0.5-1 mg/kg.

Real Health MD's Guide to Breast Surgery

The first part of the treatment plan for breast cancer is usually surgery. There are ways to optimize your body and prepare yourself for the best surgical outcome.

Here is your guide to optimal surgical outcome.

One week before:
1. Do everything you can to increase your nutrient load. Aim to eat as many colorful plants as possible. Variety is key here.

2. SKIP THE SUGAR! Sugar is immunosuppressive and adversely affects your metabolic health and your ability to fight off infection and heal.

3. Speak with your surgeon about pain control (see #2 under During Surgery).

4. Ask about supplements. I have not found supplements like fish oil or turmeric to be an issue with surgery, although they are frequently cautioned against. It is up to you whether you want to continue to use them or stop them three days prior to surgery.

5. Take 1 tablespoon of C60 twice daily one week before and one week after surgery. Then do a maintenance dose of 1 tablespoon daily. You can purchase the C60 I recommend to patients at realhealthmd.com.[29] (Note: Do not use C60 if you are getting IV Vitamin C infusions).

One day before: Fast for the whole day. Make sure you are hydrating (water, tea, broth) but skip food. We want to encourage autophagy (cell repair mode) prior to surgery.

---

[29] You can purchase C60 here: https://tinyurl.com/shopC60 .

Day of/During surgery:

1. Try to avoid the use of antibiotics. Speak with the breast surgeon, the plastic surgeon, and the anesthesiologist and share that you would prefer to not receive prophylactic (preventative) antibiotics. Breast surgery is considered a clean surgery and there is no justification or benefit to receiving antibiotics prior to your procedure. If you are having an implant placed, the plastic surgeon may insist on antibiotics. If that is the case, be sure to take a good probiotic for a month after surgery.

2. Breast surgery is rarely painful. However, the pain medicines prescribed afterward have many negative side effects ranging from constipation to immunosuppression. My patients did not use pain medicines post-op because they didn't need it. It was always my practice to inject numbing medication before I made an incision and again at the end of a procedure to keep people comfortable afterwards. Finally, for any work on the axilla (underarm where the nodes are) or when I performed a mastectomy, I always used an On-Q pump filled with bupivacaine. This device automatically delivers numbing medicine to the area for three days. It is then removed at home (it is held into place with tape). Make sure you have discussed this in advance with your surgeon and that you have a plan in place for post-op comfort and for avoiding narcotics.

After surgery:

1. All anesthetics are constipating. Be sure to have a plan in place to combat that. Have magnesium oxide or magnesium citrate at home along with Vitamin C (from ascorbic acid) to help get things going. See my guide to constipation for more details.

2. Resume your regular diet (whole food, nutrient rich, plant based, grain-free).

3. Increase your protein to 2 gm/kg/day in divided servings (kg is your weight in lbs divided by 2.2). Keep that protein level high for two weeks following the surgery. Then you can go back down to 1-1.5 gm/kg/day.

4. Following your surgery, you may resume your usual supplements immediately. During this time, I increase the dose of reishi mushroom (four capsules, twice a day) to help with healing. See the resource guide or my store (realhealthmd.com) for my recommended mushroom supplements.

5. The skin takes three weeks to heal entirely. Some people are healed sooner than that. I would wait for the skin to heal before resuming the infrared sauna. Once your bandages are off and your skin is closed on its own, you may resume the use of your infrared sauna. In the meantime, showers are perfectly fine.

Real Health MD's Guide to Constipation

Constipation is a very common problem, especially following surgery. It affects up to 20% of our population so if you are constipated, you have lots of company!

What it means to be constipated is that you are moving your bowels less than once a day. Our bodies encounter a lot of toxins each day. The way our body rids itself of toxins is mainly through stool. If you are not pooping, those toxins just get reabsorbed making you feel, well, like poop!

You may be constipated due to diet, stress, antibiotics, or from not getting enough water, fiber, or healthy fat. You could also be constipated as a result of a sedentary lifestyle. Sometimes constipation is a result of something more serious, like an under-active thyroid gland. Surgery and other stressful situations can also trigger a bout of constipation.

Some Remedies for Constipation

- A whole food, plant-based diet with an additional of 2 tablespoons ground flax seeds daily. Include healthy sources of fat, including olives, avocados, nuts and seeds daily.
- Stress Management
- Avoid antibiotics use
- Exercise daily and lead an active life
- Drink six to eight glasses of filtered water a day
- Avoid caffeine and alcohol, which can be dehydrating
- Supplements
- Probiotic (Microbiome Labs Megaspore biotic)
- Magnesium Citrate (200-1,000 mg daily)
- Vitamin C (2,000-4,000 mg daily)

Use a squatty potty. The goal is to poop at least once, but ideally two to three times a day. If you don't improve on your own after using these tools, it may be time to do more investigation. You may want to find a functional medicine doctor to work with to get to the root of your problem.

General Supplements for Breast Cancer Care

- Vitamin D
- Magnesium
- Selenium
- Folate (preferably from leafy greens)
- Probiotics (especially during chemotherapy)
- Omega-3 Fatty Acids (fish oils)
- Coenzyme Q10 (CoQ10)
- Turmeric (Curcumin)
- Melatonin
- Ginseng
- Indole-3-carbinol
- DIM
- Sulforaphane

Specific Supplements for Treatment and Recovery:

During Treatment:
- Selenium
- Probiotics
- Vitamin D
- Magnesium
- Turkey Tail Mushroom
- Reishi Mushroom
- Ashwagandha (as a chemosensitizer)
- Ginseng
- High dose pancreatic enzymes
- High dose Vitamin C (during chemo)

Post-Treatment Recovery:
- C60 (Fullerene)
- Coenzyme Q10
- Omega-3 Fatty Acids

- Turmeric
- Ginseng
- Immune Modulators and Adaptogens:
- Medicinal Mushrooms (Chaga, Turkey Tail, Agaricus, Lion's Mane, Shiitake, Cordyceps, Reishi)
- Ashwagandha
- Low Dose Naltrexone
- Mistletoe

Antioxidants and Nutrients for Radiation and Chemotherapy Support:

- Turmeric (Curcumin)
- Resveratrol
- Vitamin E
- Ginger Root
- Sulforaphane (found in broccoli sprouts, kale, cabbage)
- Chinese skullcap
- Medicinal Mushrooms (Shiitake, Maitake, Lion's Mane)
- Ginseng
- Green Tea
- Dandelion Tea
- Milk Thistle Tea
- Cilantro and Parsley Tea

Supplements Targeting Specific Cancer Types:

- **Triple Negative Breast Cancer**: DIM, Melatonin, Vitamin D & K, Turmeric, EGCG, Fasting
- **HER2 Positive Tumors:** Tocotrienols (Vitamin E forms), Sorulen, Broccoli Sprouts, Curcumin, Olive Oil, Mistletoe, Beta Glucans, Fasting

Pharmaceuticals with Off-Label Uses in Cancer Care:

- Mebendazole (anti-parasitic)
- Doxycycline

- Niclosamide (chemo and radiation sensitizer)
- Claritin (for high histamine levels)
- Tagamet
- Ivermectin (anti-parasitic with anti-cancer properties)
- Low Dose Naltrexone

Supplements that Combat the Damage of Chemotherapy

There are several supplements you can take following treatment that combat the damage of chemotherapy. These include:

- **CoQ10:** Administered following breast cancer treatment, CoQ10 was found to reduce the markers of inflammation associated with cancer development.

- **Omega 3s:** These powerful anti-inflammatories reduce the inflammatory response. However, there is also evidence that they may increase response rates to chemotherapy. They are on the after list but you should discuss with your doctor whether or not to include them DURING treatment.

- Turmeric*: Though I encourage its use in cooking, the jury is still out as to whether or not it is helpful during chemotherapy. There are in vitro and animal studies that imply that turmeric may decrease the efficacy of certain chemotherapeutic drugs. The same is not true during radiation. During radiation, there is a substantial volume of evidence that curcumin is a radiosensitizer as well as a radioprotector of several normal tissues. Therefore, I recommend turmeric during radiation and beyond.

  - *A note about turmeric and tamoxifen: Because turmeric decreases the activity of the CYP3A4 enzyme, and this enzyme is the key activator of tamoxifen, turmeric is believed to decrease the effectiveness of that drug. The same is not true for the aromatase inhibitors. This only applies to tamoxifen.

- **Acetyl-L-carnitine:** It has demonstrated effectiveness in preventing and treating diabetic neuropathy and thus was of interest to help reverse chemotherapy-induced peripheral neuropathy (CIPN).

- **Lion's Mane Mushroom:** This medicinal mushroom, available as both a culinary delight and a supplement, is best known for its effect on the central nervous system. It can help to alleviate many of the residual side effects to the central nervous system caused by breast cancer treatment.

Nutrients to Consume Daily During Treatment

These are the nutrients known to protect your body from the damaging effects of radiation and chemotherapy. They also have potent anti-cancer properties. It is important to consume these in your diet while you are undergoing treatment to protect you against the negative side effects of treatment and make the treatments more effective:

- Turmeric (ground spice or root)
- Resveratrol (red grapes, pistachios, blueberries, bilberries, cacao)
- Vitamin E (almonds, peanuts, hazelnuts, spinach, broccoli)
- Ginger root or ground ginger
- Sulforaphane (broccoli sprouts, broccoli, kale, cabbage, watercress)
- Medicinal mushrooms (shiitake, maitake, lion's mane)
- Green Tea
- Dandelion tea
- Milk thistle tea
- Cilantro and Parsley tea (can be combined)

Radiation Protection Protocol

This radiation protection protocol. This should be used the day prior to your study, one hour prior to your study, and for three days following your study. For X Rays, CT scans, bone scans, PET scans, DEXA scans, mammograms, or any study that involves ionizing radiation (exceptions are ultrasound or MRI), this protocol should be followed.

Melatonin 20 mg, once per day: Take 100-300mg (5-15 capsules) one hour prior to radiologic study. If you are worried about sedation, do a trial run prior to see how you respond. This is not a sleep dose.

Liposomal Vitamin C: Take 2-4 tsp (2000-4000mg) one day before your study, then one hour prior, and for three days following your radiologic study. Warning, vitamin C at this dose may give you diarrhea or loose stools.

Nanoemulsified D3K2, once per day: Take eight pumps daily BEFORE 3:00pm starting the day before your study and continue for three days following your study. Hold under tongue for 30 seconds before swallowing. (Five days total).

Liposomal Glutathione, 2 pumps twice per day: Take two pumps daily starting the day before your study and continue for three days following your study. Hold under tongue for 30 seconds before swallowing (Five days total). Best taken on an empty stomach.

Ultra Pure® Fish Oil, 1 gel, twice per day: Take one gel twice daily starting the day before your study and continue for three days following your study. (Five days total). Best taken with food.

To access the radiation protection protocol and supplements, scan the QR code on page 207.

MRI Protection Protocol

If you are undergoing an MRI with gadolinium (contrast), gadolinium is a heavy metal which gets absorbed in your bloodstream and stored in the tissues of your body. Anytime we store heavy metals in the body we do that at the expense of something we need.

You can use this protocol to minimize the amount of gadolinium you uptake and therefore decrease the likelihood of permanent damage.

The best way to avoid injury from MRI is not to use it. I do not recommend using MRI for screening purposes. If you need it to help with diagnosis, follow this protocol.

You will be taking zinc for five days starting the day before your study and continuing for three days after your study (including the day of your study).

Adequate levels of zinc will prevent gadolinium absorption. I have included two forms of zinc as they are the ones best absorbed. Take BOTH of them. Do not supplement with zinc long term as it will lead to malabsorption of other vital nutrients.

- Zinc Bisglycinate 15mg - Take two capsule daily for five days starting the day before your MRI. Take with food. Be sure to take the zinc at least one hour prior to your MRI on the day of your study.
- Zinc Picolinate 30 mg - 180 Capsules - Take one capsule daily for five days starting the day before your MRI. Take with food. Be sure to take the zinc at least one hour prior to your MRI on the day of your study.

To access the MRI protection protocol and supplements, scan the QR code on page 207.

Daily Eight Guide

Incorporate the Daily Eight into your nutrition plan to drastically improve your diet, health, and inflammatory response.

- Green Tea: consume four cups of green tea a day.
- Garlic: Incorporate into meals daily.
- Brazil nuts: Four a day for your daily dose of selenium.
- Flax Seed: Two tablespoons per day of ground flax seed.
- Cruciferous: Include broccoli, broccoli sprouts, cauliflower, brussel sprouts, cabbage bok choy.
- Mushrooms: Culinary mushrooms are shitake, maitake, and lion's mane. These are the most potent, but all mushrooms have aromatase inhibiting properties and help with hormone balance.
- Onion Family: Onion, shallots, fennel, and leek.

You should have healthy fat at every meal. Those include olive oil, avocado oil, avocados, coconut oil, olives, nuts, and seeds.

Over the course of the week, try to make sure you are consuming vegetables across the phytonutrient spectrum (all the colors). Overall, your goal is to consume 6-9 cups of non-starchy vegetables a day. These are your daily basics. Concentrate on 75% of your plate being non-starchy colorful vegetables.

Weekly Checklist

All of these foods should be non-GMO and organic.

Healthy Fats
Almonds, avocado Oil, avocados, brazil nuts, flax seeds, ground flaxseeds, hazelnuts, hemp seeds, nut butters, olives, olive oil, pecans, pine nuts, pistachio nuts, pumpkin seeds, sesame seeds, sesame seed oil, sunflowers, walnuts.

Proteins
Beans, legumes, tofu, tempeh, chickpeas, lentils, navy beans, cannellini beans, nuts (also under fats), wild caught fish, wild caught shellfish, pasture raised poultry, pasture raised eggs, grass fed beef, grass fed wild game, organ meats.

Note: If you choose to include animal products, consume no more than one fist sized serving per day.

Vegetables
Brussels Sprouts, cabbage, kale, broccoli, carrots, peppers, celery, cabbages, spinach, asparagus, okra, broccoli sprouts, watercress, collard greens, mustard greens, fennel, shallots, beet greens, beets, scallions, artichoke, mushrooms, red onion, shallots, tomatoes.

Fruits
Green Apples. Red apples, cherries, citrus fruits, lemons and limes, blueberries, cranberries, bilberries, strawberries, blackberries, black raspberries, guava, kiwi, papaya.

Spices and Herbs
Garlic, onion, oregano, sage, thyme, parsley, basil, stinging nettle root, dandelion greens and root, marjoram, lavender, hawthorn leaves and

flowers, turmeric, ginger, fennel, rosemary, cilantro, cumin, coriander, horseradish, capsaicin (hot pepper).

Medicinal Mushrooms
Turkey Tail, Reishi, Cordyceps, Chaga, Shitake, Maitake Lions Mane.

YES AND NO LIST

YES:

- Non-starchy vegetables
- Berries (organic, a cup a day)
- Nuts and Seeds
- Olives (unless you are salt sensitive)
- Unsweetened and gum free nut milks and nutbutters
- Legumes & Beans
- Healthy fats: olive oil, avocado oil (good for cooking), avocados, and coconut oil
- Fruit (beyond your essential berries) should be limited to 1-2 servings a day, should be organic, seasonal, and should not be used as a substitute for eating your vegetables.

NO:

- Sugar or sugar substitutes
- Processed grains: (flour, bread, crackers, pasta, cereal, cake, and cookies)
- Juice
- Soft drinks
- GMO products: corn, soy, and wheat
- Gluten
- Bacon, Sausage, Hot dogs, Pork Roll, Deli Meat, Beef, chicken, pork or other factory farm meats
- Farm raised fish or shellfish

- Processed oils: corn, soybean, canola (rapeseed), safflower, vegetable, sunflower, peanut, cottonseed, rice bran, grapeseed.
- Trans fats: margarine, butter substitutes
- Grains: even whole grains
- Dairy: milk, cream, butter, cheese, yogurt.
    - *Remember all animal products, even humanely raised animal products, are pro-growth and contribute to the development of cancer.*

ABOUT THE AUTHOR

Dr. Jenn Simmons is an Integrative Oncologist, Breast Surgeon, Author, Podcast Host, and the founder of PerfeQTion Imaging. Her journey into breast cancer care began with a personal tragedy. At the age of 16, Dr. Jenn's cousin, acclaimed singer-songwriter Linda Creed, died of metastatic breast cancer just weeks after Whitney Houston's recording of her iconic song, "The Greatest Love of All," topped the charts. This loss became a defining moment, inspiring Dr. Jenn to dedicate her life to transforming how we approach breast cancer treatment and prevention.

Dr. Jenn became Philadelphia's first fellowship-trained breast surgeon and spent 17 years leading the field. However, her perspective changed significantly when she became a patient herself. Through this personal experience, Dr. Jenn saw how broken the conventional medical system can be. This led her to discover and embrace functional medicine, a revelation that sparked her journey towards a more holistic approach to breast cancer care.

This personal journey led her to create Real Health MD in 2019, a practice dedicated to holistic healing for breast cancer. It integrates conventional wisdom with root cause medicine and the drivers of health: nutrition, lifestyle changes, detoxification, and stress management. Dr. Jenn's innovative approach doesn't stop there. As the founder of PerfeQTion Imaging, she is establishing safe imaging centers across the nation, armed with revolutionary technology that promises to redefine breast cancer screening. This technology is not only fast and safe but also comfortable, affordable, radiation-free, and boasts 40 times the resolution of MRI. It has received FDA clearance, signaling a new era in breast health and breast cancer screening.

In addition to her clinical practice, Dr. Jenn hosts the "Keeping Abreast" podcast, where she shares her expertise and encourages women to take control of their breast health. Her book, "The Smart Woman's Guide to Breast Cancer," challenges conventional wisdom and promotes a holistic approach. It emphasizes the importance of nutrition, lifestyle choices, and addressing environmental toxins, providing practical steps for women seeking to navigate breast cancer treatment and regain control of their health.

Beyond her professional endeavors, Dr. Jenn is a devoted wife, mother, stepmother, grandmother, and athlete. Her life's mission is deeply personal, rooted in her cousin's memory, and driven by a desire to make a lasting impact on all those who desire breast health. As she famously says, "Breast Health is Health!

Made in the USA
Columbia, SC
21 November 2024

47202987R00133